Adapting Your Home: Simple Changes to Reduce Arthritis Risk

By LA Smith

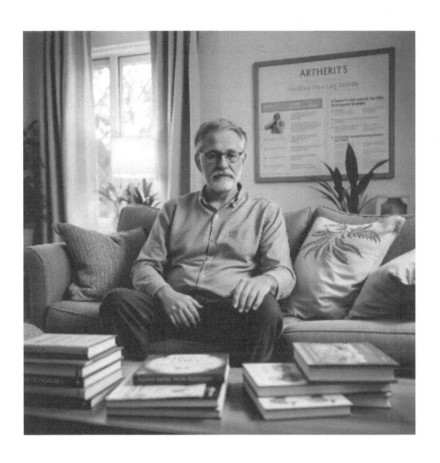

Disclaimer

The information provided in *Adapting Your Home: Simple Changes to Reduce Arthritis Risk* is for educational and informational purposes only. It is not intended as medical, legal, or professional advice and should not be used as a substitute for consultation with qualified healthcare professionals, occupational therapists, or home safety specialists. Readers should consult with their physician or other healthcare providers before making any changes to their home, lifestyle, or treatment plans.

While every effort has been made to ensure the accuracy and reliability of the content, LA Smith and LA Smith Publishing make no representations or warranties, express or implied, regarding the completeness, accuracy, or applicability of the information contained within this book. The authors and publishers shall not be held liable for any loss, injury, or damages—direct or indirect—that may result from the use of this book.

Some recommendations in this book may not be suitable for all individuals or home environments. Readers are encouraged to conduct their own research and seek professional guidance to determine what modifications best suit their needs and circumstances.

By reading this book, you acknowledge that you assume full responsibility for any actions taken based on the information provided.

About
LA Smith is a dedicated researcher and advocate for those affected by arthritis, driven by a deep-seated passion to improve the lives of men and women living with this condition. With years of in-depth study on adaptive home solutions, Smith combines personal experience with professional expertise to offer practical advice that empowers individuals to minimize their arthritis risk. LA Smith is commitment to fostering healthier living environments shines through in every page.

Table of Contents

7

Chapter 1: Understanding Arthritis

What is Arthritis?

Arthritis is more than just a medical term; it's a daily reality for millions of men and women, transforming how they navigate their lives. At its core, arthritis refers to the inflammation of the joints, which can lead to pain, stiffness, and swelling, making even the simplest tasks feel like monumental challenges. Picture waking up in the morning, and as you reach for your cup of coffee, a sharp pain flares up in your hands. This isn't just a fleeting discomfort; it's the manifestation of a condition that can affect every aspect of your daily routine. With over 100 different types of arthritis, ranging from osteoarthritis, which often comes with age, to rheumatoid arthritis, an autoimmune disorder, it's crucial to understand that each person's experience can vary dramatically. As the joints become inflamed, mobility can diminish, and what once seemed effortless can transform into an uphill battle.

Understanding arthritis is essential, not only for those living with the condition but also for loved ones and caregivers who support them. By fostering empathy towards those who experience joint pain, we can create a more compassionate world. Awareness of the condition helps in making lifestyle changes that can provide relief and improve quality of life. This may include simple adjustments, such as choosing supportive footwear or engaging in gentle exercises. It also involves recognizing the emotional toll that arthritis has on individuals. Many carry the weight of frustration and sadness as they confront limitations on their physical capabilities. Acknowledging this emotional landscape not only benefits those affected but also encourages a supportive environment, fostering connections and understanding among friends and family. Small acts of kindness, like offering to assist with chores or simply listening, can make a world of difference.

It's important to remember that living with arthritis doesn't mean losing your zest for life. Finding coping strategies, including staying informed about managing the condition and connecting with support networks, can empower you. Seek out resources that provide helpful tips, such as engaging in low-impact activities like swimming or yoga, which can aid in managing symptoms without placing too much strain on the joints. Each step you take, no matter how small, contributes to a healthier, more fulfilled life. Consider talking to your healthcare provider about a personalized plan that supports both your physical and emotional well-being, ensuring that arthritis remains a part of your story without defining it.

Types of Arthritis

Arthritis is a term that covers a wide range of conditions affecting the joints. The differences between these types are significant, as they can dictate the pain levels, the management plans, and our everyday lives. Osteoarthritis is one of the most common forms, arising from wear and tear on the joints over the years. This degenerative condition can lead to stiffness and inflammation, often making simple tasks like climbing stairs or picking up objects feel like a monumental effort. It primarily affects older adults, but younger individuals are not exempt, especially if they've suffered joint injuries or have certain risk factors like obesity.

On the other hand, rheumatoid arthritis is an autoimmune condition that can affect anyone at any age. When I first learned about it, I was shocked to discover that it doesn't just attack the joints; it can impact the body as a whole. The immune system mistakenly attacks the synovium—the lining of the membranes that surround joints. This can lead to painful swelling, reduced mobility, and sometimes even structural damage to the joints if left untreated. Understanding these differences brings a sense of clarity, especially for anyone struggling with joint pain. The emotional toll of arthritis is significant. Learning about different types can feel empowering rather than isolating, allowing you to seek the specific care that you need.

Recognizing the unique characteristics of each type can tailor your approach to prevention and management, helping you live a more vibrant life despite the challenges. For example, if you know you are dealing with osteoarthritis, strengthening the muscles surrounding your joints can provide greater support and alleviate some of the pressure. Engaging in low-impact exercises like swimming or biking can keep you mobile. Meanwhile, for someone with rheumatoid arthritis, working closely with a rheumatologist to manage inflammation through medication and lifestyle changes can make all the difference. We all want to feel heard and understood, and knowing the specific type of arthritis empowers us to communicate better with our healthcare providers and develop a personalized plan. It might be helpful to keep a journal of your symptoms to discuss during your appointments. Documenting how different movements feel or noting when the pain worsens can lead to more tailored advice. Finding effective strategies is not just about managing symptoms; it's about reclaiming our lives.

Symptoms and Diagnosis

Arthritis can manifest in various ways, and recognizing its common signs and symptoms is crucial for timely action. Many individuals experience swelling or tenderness in their joints, which may gradually develop or arrive suddenly. Stiffness, especially in the morning or after sitting for long periods, can make daily activities challenging. It's not uncommon to feel a persistent ache or pain in the affected areas, which may worsen with movement or during certain weather conditions. Some might notice a decrease in their range of motion, feeling as though their joints are tighter or less flexible than before. Fatigue is another alarming symptom that can accompany joint issues, leaving you feeling exhausted even after a good night's sleep. Additionally, a general sense of malaise or fever can be experienced, suggesting that something is not quite right within the body. Being attuned to these symptoms enables individuals to take control and seek help sooner rather than later.

Understanding how arthritis is diagnosed is essential for early intervention and effective management. Typically, the journey begins with a thorough evaluation by a healthcare professional who will assess your symptom history and perform a physical examination. Imaging tests, such as X-rays or MRI scans, can provide vital insight into joint damage or inflammation, helping to clarify the diagnosis. Further, blood tests may be conducted to check for specific

14

markers that indicate certain types of arthritis, such as rheumatoid arthritis. The process may seem overwhelming, but each step is a critical part of the puzzle that leads to a clearer understanding of your condition. Early detection is key; it sets the stage for more effective treatment options that can help to slow down the progression of the disease. Recognizing the symptoms and moving forward with the diagnostic process empowers you to manage your arthritis better.

Awareness of your body and the changes you experience is vital in navigating life with arthritis. Many people find it helpful to keep a journal of their symptoms, noting when they occur and any potential triggers. This practice not only aids in recognizing patterns but can also provide your healthcare provider with useful information for diagnosis and treatment planning. Listening to your body, advocating for yourself during medical appointments, and seeking the knowledge you need are your allies in this journey.

Impact on Daily Life

Living with arthritis often reshapes not just the body, but also the entire landscape of daily activities and quality of life. For many, simple tasks that once felt effortless can become monumental challenges. You may find that getting out of bed in the morning is no longer an automatic action; the stiffness and pain can make you reconsider even the most basic movements. Everyday activities like tying your shoes, cooking dinner, or even holding a cup of coffee can turn into battles, causing frustration and fatigue. This struggle doesn't go unnoticed—it wears away at your sense of independence and often leads to feelings of isolation. As you navigate your day, you may start to avoid activities you once enjoyed for fear of triggering pain or discomfort, which can gradually diminish your overall well-being and happiness.

Real stories shed light on the emotional journey of those living with arthritis. Susan, a vibrant woman in her 40s, shares how her diagnosis transformed her identity. I used to love gardening. The feel of soil in my hands and the joy of nurturing plants brought me peace, she recounts, her voice heavy with emotion. Now, just bending down to pull weeds feels like a Herculean task. I often sit on the porch, watching the flowers bloom from afar. It breaks my heart. Similarly, James, a retired teacher in his 60s, expresses the frustration of canceling plans with friends. It's like a shadow follows me wherever I go, he explains. The thought of using a cane at his age feels like a defeat, driving a wedge between him and his social life. Both stories highlight the unspoken emotional toll of arthritis—how it isolates and diminishes the spirit, and how laughter, often your best medicine, becomes harder to come by.

Finding ways to cope can make a significant difference. Remember, you're not alone in this journey. Many people are going through similar struggles, and sharing your experiences can foster connection and support. Consider joining a local support group or an online community where stories and strategies are exchanged. Whether it's discovering tools that can help ease daily tasks, or simply having a place to talk about the highs and lows, staying connected to others who understand can empower you to reclaim joy in your life.

Importance of Lifestyle Changes

Making lifestyle changes can significantly reduce arthritis symptoms and enhance overall well-being. Every small adjustment to your daily routine can create waves of positive impact. For instance, incorporating gentle exercises like swimming or yoga can improve flexibility and strengthen muscles, providing relief from pain. It's important to focus on your diet too; eating anti-inflammatory foods such as leafy greens, nuts, and fatty fish can help to reduce swelling and discomfort. Staying hydrated is equally vital, as it can help maintain joint lubrication and overall cellular function. I remember when I began to notice my own stubbornness about these changes. It was a slow journey, but each step made me feel more empowered and resilient against the grip of arthritis.

Taking proactive steps in managing arthritis means embracing choices that can change your life for the better. It's easy to feel overwhelmed, but breaking these changes into manageable bits can make a difference. Instead of aiming for perfection, just focus on consistency. Substitute a few processed snacks with options that nurture your body. Plan your day to include short walks, allowing your joints to benefit without overexerting yourself. It may feel daunting at first, but each thoughtful choice builds a new habit. Connect with others who share similar experiences; support can motivate you to persist. Remember that every positive change you make today lays down the foundation for a better tomorrow. Consider journaling your journey, noting not only the changes you make but also how they help you feel, which can be incredibly rewarding and encouraging as you track your progress.

A simple yet powerful practice is setting aside a few minutes each day for mindfulness. This could mean meditative breathing or simply being present with your thoughts. Stress can trigger flare-ups, so finding moments of peace is vital. You deserve to feel good in your body. Embrace these changes, knowing that each step, small or large, is a step toward a healthier, more fulfilling life.

Chapter 2: The Role of Home Environment

How Environment Affects Arthritis

Your home environment plays a critical role in managing arthritis symptoms, often acting as a double-edged sword. For many of us living with this condition, the spaces we inhabit can either bring relief or exacerbate our pain. Consider the design and layout of your home. Open spaces with plenty of natural light can provide a sense of calm and comfort that may lessen the stress on your joints, while cluttered areas may lead to unexpected falls or excessive bending and stretching, triggering unwanted pain. Simple adjustments, such as ensuring that frequently used items are within easy reach or using supportive furniture, can transform a space and significantly impact day-to-day comfort. Also, the indoor climate matters. Keeping your home at a stable, moderate temperature can help manage stiffness; using humidifiers can alleviate dry air and make breathing easier, contributing to overall wellness and reducing stress on your body.

Understanding the connection between comfort, safety, and joint health is fundamental for anyone managing arthritis. A home that feels safe can bring immense peace of mind, allowing you to move with less anxiety about falling or injuring yourself. Non-slip rugs, stable handrails, and well-lit areas contribute significantly to creating a secure space where you can relax. This enables you to focus on your hobbies and engage in gentle activities that promote joint flexibility and strength, rather than worrying about potential hazards. Moreover, comfort goes beyond physical safety; it also encompasses emotional well-being. Surrounding yourself with items that inspire joy and calm - whether it's family photos, artwork, or plants - can uplift your mood and, in turn, positively impact your physical health. This holistic approach to your environment engages the body and mind, helping you remain positive in the face of the challenges that arthritis brings.

Common Home Hazards

Everyday life can create a myriad of hazards, especially for those living with arthritis. Navigating your home should be a comforting experience, but sometimes even the slightest things can trigger pain or discomfort. It's essential to recognize the common hazards that can turn a simple task into a daunting challenge. Areas like the bathroom can pose significant risks with slippery surfaces, making it hard to maintain balance. Kitchen drawers that stick or cabinets placed too high can lead to frustration and potential falls. Even the layout of your furniture can become an obstacle; tight spaces can make it difficult to move freely, increasing the risk of bumping into hard edges, leading not just to discomfort but also injury. Being mindful of these everyday hazards not only enhances safety but also preserves your independence.

Awareness of potential hazards is the first step towards creating a safer home environment. By understanding where risks are likely to occur, you can take proactive measures to protect yourself. Simple changes can make a world of difference; for example, installing grab bars in the bathroom or non-slip mats in the shower can greatly reduce the chances of falling. Rearranging furniture to create clearer pathways allows for smoother navigation around the house, easing physical strain. Using tools designed for ease, such as jar openers or long-handled reachers, can minimize the need to bend or twist in ways that may cause discomfort. Consider the importance of proper lighting as well; brightening up dimly lit areas can help spot obstacles and reduce missteps, helping to maintain your confidence at home.

Taking time to assess your living space can lead to significant improvements in your day-to-day life. Small adjustments can provide peace of mind, knowing you've taken steps towards a safer home. Remember, each positive change you make contributes to a more supportive environment, helping you to live life to the fullest even with arthritis. Consider creating a checklist of potential hazards and prioritize what changes will have the greatest impact on your safety and comfort. This proactive approach not only empowers you but fosters a sense of control over your living space.

Identifying Risk Zones

Pinpointing areas in your home that may pose increased risks for injury is an important step in creating a safer environment. As someone who has taken the time to assess my own living space, I've realized that many accidents can be traced back to overlooked hazards in those everyday corners that we often dismiss. Start by walking through each room with a critical eye. Look for loose rugs that might trip you up, poorly placed furniture that narrows pathways, or clutter that leaves little room to maneuver. Think about your daily routines and consider the moments when you might feel rushed or distracted. These moments can lead to missteps, and addressing potential hazards can make a significant difference. Pay special attention to commonly used areas, like the kitchen and bathroom, where slips and falls are more likely to occur. Installing non-slip mats or adding grab bars can significantly enhance safety in these risk zones.

Assessing your space safely and effectively requires a thoughtful approach. Engage with your surroundings and take notes on what feels safe and what does not. Are there areas where lighting is inadequate, making nighttime navigation treacherous? If you have a basement or attic, evaluate the stairs' condition and ensure proper lighting is installed. To create a truly safe haven, consider inviting friends or family to help share their perspectives; often, a fresh set of eyes can grab our attention to potential risks we might overlook. Don't hesitate to ask for feedback on how user-friendly your space is for everyone. Sometimes, small adjustments like moving a chair or lowering a shelf can enhance accessibility and reduce the likelihood of accidents.

Remember, making your home a safer haven is about creating an environment that promotes confidence in daily activities. One practical tip is to perform regular safety audits. Set aside a certain day each month to review your living space, making note of any new hazards that may have crept in. You could even keep a checklist to track the adjustments you've made over time, which can motivate you to stay proactive. Ultimately, the goal is to establish a secure space where you and your loved ones can thrive, free from unnecessary worry about trips and falls.

Creating a Safe Space

Transforming your home into a comfortable and safe living environment starts with understanding your space and its layout. Begin by taking a good look around your home and identifying areas that feel cluttered or chaotic. These spaces can often evoke stress and anxiety. Clear out items that no longer serve a purpose or bring you joy. Having a minimalist approach often leads to a more welcoming atmosphere. Consider investing in storage solutions that not only enhance organization but also blend harmoniously with your decor. For example, decorative bins and shelves can keep your belongings tucked away while still being aesthetically pleasing. Additionally, soft lighting can create a warm and inviting ambiance. Opt for lamps with dimmers or warm bulbs to help you sink into a cozy, relaxed state after a long day.

The psychological benefits of living in a well-organized, hazard-free home cannot be understated. An orderly environment fosters a sense of calm. When your surroundings are manageable, it's easier to focus on your mental and emotional well-being. Studies have shown that clutter can amplify feelings of anxiety, so decluttering can be a powerful first step toward achieving tranquility. Picture coming home to a space where everything has its place—the color scheme is soothing, and the air feels fresh. This reality allows your mind to escape daily stresses, creating a sanctuary that nurtures rather than drains you. Establishing areas dedicated to relaxation—whether it's a reading nook with comforting cushions or a meditation corner—can significantly enhance your emotional landscape, offering you a retreat from the outside world.

One practical tip is to regularly assess your space. Take a moment each week to notice anything that feels out of place or cluttered, and address it immediately. This regular check-in not only keeps your environment thriving but also ensures that small annoyances do not accumulate into larger stressors. By creating a habit of nurturing your home, you empower yourself to maintain a safe, inviting space that supports and uplifts you.

Psychological Effects of Environment

A supportive and safe environment has the power to uplift and nurture our mental health. It creates a space where we can express ourselves freely, where we feel heard and valued. When surrounded by understanding friends, family, or even co-workers, we begin to feel a sense of belonging. This feeling is essential; it fosters resilience and encourages us to tackle life's challenges with a more optimistic mindset. Each interaction in these safe spaces reinforces our sense of self-worth and can significantly reduce feelings of anxiety and depression. I recall moments spent in warm, inviting settings—be it the gentle embrace of loved ones, the tranquility of nature, or even a favorite coffee shop bustling with life. Such spaces transform and rejuvenate us, reminding us that we are not alone in our struggles. It's like filling an empty cup with warmth; suddenly, what seemed impossible becomes manageable.

Understanding the importance of our environments offers each of us a unique opportunity. It invites us to assess our own spaces and make conscious choices that would enhance our lives. Small changes, like decluttering a room, introducing plants, or creating an inspiring corner for mindful practices, can significantly impact our mood and motivation. Let's not underestimate the power of a well-placed plant or a favorite photograph—these little details can evoke happiness and spark creativity. Cultivating a personal sanctuary, no matter how small, can provide a sense of peace in the chaos of daily life. As you navigate through your living or working spaces, remember: these environments are an extension of you. Curate them wisely, and you may just unveil a brighter perspective on life.

Chapter 3: Ergonomic Design Principles

The Basics of Ergonomics

Understanding ergonomic principles is vital, especially for individuals living with arthritis. These principles focus on designing workspaces and tasks that accommodate our bodies' natural position and movements, reducing strain and pain. For those of us who face daily challenges with joint discomfort, ergonomics can feel like a lifeline. Every small adjustment that promotes better posture, reduces pressure on our joints, and fosters a more natural range of motion can make a significant difference. Imagine how transforming your workstation or the way you perform daily tasks could alleviate some of the constant aches. Simple things like adjusting your chair height or changing the way you lift objects can create a ripple effect in your quality of life. These adjustments are not just about comfort; they can be empowering, giving us a sense of control over our health amidst the unpredictability of arthritis.

Ergonomics can actively enhance both comfort and mobility, especially when arthritis tends to limit our movements. It encourages us to listen to our bodies and respond proactively. For instance, consider how modifying the usage of tools can lighten the strain on our hands and joints. Choosing ergonomic utensils with soft grips or wider handles can make mundane tasks, such as cooking or cleaning, less painful and more manageable. Additionally, arranging your home or workspace to minimize reaching, bending, or twisting can open up new avenues for mobility. When we learn to create environments that cater to our specific needs, we allow ourselves to move freely without fear of exacerbating pain. The feeling of getting through daily tasks with greater ease can uplift our spirits and inspire us to stay active longer.

Implementing ergonomic strategies does not have to be overwhelming. Start with one small change—perhaps adjust your chair to better support your back while sitting. Observe how this shift impacts your comfort levels during the day. As you become more aware of your body's needs, you may find it easier to identify additional changes that can enhance your life. Seek out resources like adaptive tools designed specifically for individuals with arthritis, which can further facilitate smoother movements. Remember, every effort counts, and even minor adjustments can lead to significant improvements in your daily life.

Furniture Choices for Comfort

Selecting ergonomic furniture is crucial for anyone who values comfort, especially those of us with physical sensitivities or joint concerns. I've often found myself overwhelmed by choices in stores, yet understanding the importance of ergonomics drastically changed that experience for me. Ergonomic furniture is designed to support the natural posture of your body. The key is to look for pieces that provide ample support while reducing strain on your joints. This means finding chairs with the right height, depth, and back support that align with your body's unique needs. I remember the first time I sat in a chair that cradled my lower back; the relief was immediate and undeniable. Your goal should be to create a space where your body feels at ease, allowing you to focus on your tasks without the distraction of discomfort.

When considering helpful features, height adjustability and lumbar support stand out as invaluable investments. A chair that adjusts to your height can prevent unnecessary strain on your knees and hips, allowing your feet to rest comfortably on the ground. I discovered that having this flexibility transformed not just my comfort level but also my productivity. Equally important is lumbar support, which helps maintain the natural curve of your spine. Many chairs come with adjustable lumbar features that enable you to customize the support to fit your back precisely. Investing in a desk that allows you to alternate between sitting and standing can also be a game-changer. Not only does it promote better posture, but it also encourages movement throughout the day, which I've found tremendously beneficial for my energy levels.

Ultimately, the right furniture goes beyond aesthetics; it should feel like a sanctuary for your body. Always try out furniture before buying it, if possible. Spend a few minutes sitting on a chair or adjusting a desk to see how it feels. Your body will let you know if it's a good fit or not. Choosing the right ergonomic furniture can be one of the best decisions for your well-being, relieving pressure and allowing you to enjoy your activities without physical limitations.

Placement of Objects for Accessibility

Arranging furniture and items in a way that minimizes unnecessary physical strain can transform your living space into a sanctuary of comfort. Consider the journey you take daily through your home — the way you reach for items, the twists and turns you navigate. When placing furniture, think about creating clear pathways. Aim for spaces that feel open, allowing you to move without effort. For example, if your kitchen cabinets are filled with frequently used spices or utensils, position them within easy reach, perhaps at waist level rather than high above. This minor adjustment may drastically reduce the risk of strain or injury while cooking. Also, ensure that furniture corners are rounded or protected to prevent any accidents that could disturb the equilibrium of your routine. Take into account your physical needs and the particular demands of the tasks you undertake, allowing yourself room to breathe as you move. The way you arrange your space should serve you, not hinder your daily activities.

Creating ease of access tailored to your daily needs allows for a more fluid and enjoyable lifestyle. It's important to audit your environment regularly, assessing which items you use most frequently and adjusting their placement accordingly. For instance, if you often find yourself reaching for items on a shelf that feels too high, consider relocating those items to a lower shelf or utilizing pull-out drawers. Think about all the little moments — the coffee cup you grab every morning or the shoes you put on as you head out. By ensuring everything is within easy reach, you empower yourself to move through your day without struggle. You might also explore the concept of zoning your space; for instance, keep clutter-free areas for relaxation, separate from activity zones. This not only promotes accessibility but nurtures a state of mind that fosters productivity and peace.

Another practical consideration is lighting; ensure that areas where you engage in tasks are well-lit, reducing the need to strain your eyes while searching for objects. It's a simple yet profound way to enhance accessibility and comfort. By creating a space that acknowledges your needs and preferences, you're not just making life easier; you're cultivating an environment that respects your energy and well-being. Remember, the goal is to eliminate barriers, even the smallest ones. Begin with one area of your home and pay attention to how these adjustments make you feel. Each thoughtful change allows you to reclaim your space bit by bit, leading to a home that truly supports you in every aspect.

Adjustable Features in Your Home

Adjustable furniture and fixtures can truly transform a living space, especially for those of us managing arthritis. These pieces not only prioritize comfort but also enhance accessibility, allowing you to move freely without the struggle that often comes with traditional, static furniture. Imagine a dining table that can change height, accommodating not just your needs but also the needs of guests. Or a bed that can be easily adjusted for a more comfortable position at night, reducing stress on your joints. The ability to modify these elements to suit your daily routine can lead to a remarkable improvement in the quality of life. It's all about creating an environment that respects your limitations while celebrating your independence.

Flexibility and adaptability have become crucial components of a supportive home, particularly when managing a condition like arthritis. Your home should evolve with you, allowing you to live comfortably and confidently. Adjustable features in your environment mean that you are not confined by your condition; rather, you can shape your surroundings to meet your ongoing needs. Consider how easy it is to use a chair that adjusts to the perfect height, providing support when standing or sitting down. Every adjustment you make is a step towards a more inclusive and understanding space that encourages you to engage with your home fully.

Choosing adjustable options doesn't just cater to your physical needs; they also provide emotional comfort. Having a home that feels accommodating can reduce feelings of frustration and helplessness. It empowers you to take control of your living space in a way that leads to well-being and peace of mind. Remember, the smallest changes can create significant impacts. Start by evaluating your current furniture and consider what adjustments could make a real difference in your daily routine. Investing in adjustable features is not just about comfort; it's about reclaiming your space and your independence.

Importance of Ergonomic Tools

Dealing with arthritis can feel like an uphill battle, especially in the midst of everyday tasks that once seemed second nature. Simple actions such as opening a jar or writing a note can become daunting challenges. However, ergonomic tools can profoundly impact our daily experiences, making our lives easier and more comfortable. Designed with the human body in mind, these tools help reduce strain on our joints and improve our grip. For instance, ergonomically designed kitchen utensils with soft, cushioned handles not only make cooking more enjoyable but also alleviate discomfort while preparing meals. This can transform cooking from a chore into a pleasurable activity.

Consider the role of ergonomic office chairs and desks for those who spend long hours at a computer. These equipped workspaces can be adjusted for optimal posture, reducing stiffness and pain in the shoulders and back. The right setup allows individuals to work effectively while minimizing the physical toll that arthritis can take. Even simple devices, like jar openers and button hooks, can restore independence. All these tools work towards creating a more harmonious interaction with the world around us, enabling you to handle activities of daily living with increased confidence and ease.

Investing in ergonomic tools and modifications may feel like a significant step, but it is crucial for maintaining quality of life. Every purchase is an investment in comfort and independence. You don't have to push through pain or discomfort while attempting tasks that, while important, should not require a toll on your physical wellbeing. By prioritizing ergonomic adaptations, you enable yourself to reclaim joy in the little things that make life rich. It's about finding solutions that work best for you, whether that means equipping your home with special aids or simply rearranging furniture to suit your needs better.

Take the plunge and assess your environment—what changes can you implement today to reduce strain? Perhaps an adjustable bed can facilitate restful sleep, or a reacher tool can help you grasp items without bending to the floor. As you make these modifications, remember that the goal is not just comfort but a renewed sense of empowerment. Each upgrade is a step towards embracing your abilities rather than feeling hindered by limitations. Therefore, reflect on your daily activities and consider how even the smallest ergonomic solutions can improve your functionality and overall comfort.

If you're unsure where to start, think about your most challenging tasks and explore available ergonomic options designed specifically for those needs. A small investment can yield significant benefits, helping you live a more fulfilling life with greater ease.

Chapter 4: Flooring Solutions

Best Flooring Options for Arthritis

When living with arthritis, one of the essential changes can be found underfoot. The choice of flooring plays a vital role in how comfortable your surroundings feel. Soft, cushioned materials such as cork or carpet can provide a welcoming underfoot experience that eases pressure on joints. Cork, in particular, offers a combination of durability and warmth, making it easy on the feet while reducing impact when walking. Carpets can be inviting, but be mindful of their thickness; a more plush carpet might trap dirt and make it difficult to walk on safely. Vinyl and laminate flooring can also be great options, as they combine easy maintenance with a level of softness that can help reduce discomfort. Both materials provide a smooth surface, which makes transitions from one area to another easier on sore joints and can also accommodate assistive devices if needed.

Selecting the right flooring isn't just about aesthetics; it's about creating a space that minimizes stress on your joints. Taking into account the maintenance, slip-resistant surfaces, and ease of cleaning can make a significant difference in daily life. Ensure that any flooring you consider has a texture that provides grip, reducing the risk of falls, which can be particularly concerning for those with arthritis. It's also worthwhile to consider the temperature of the flooring material; some can feel cold underfoot, which can be uncomfortable for sensitive joints. Using area rugs in key locations can add warmth and comfort, providing additional cushioning where you stand most. Remember, your environment should empower you, not hinder your mobility, and prioritizing slip resistance and cushioned comfort can enhance your quality of life.

One practical tip is to choose flooring that allows for easy maintenance; the less time you spend on your feet cleaning, the better. Look for options that are easy to wipe down or resistant to stains, and consider getting a vacuum cleaner or a mop that's lightweight and easy to maneuver. This simple adjustment can make day-to-day tasks less taxing on your body. Don't hesitate to visualize how each option could fit into your lifestyle and the comfort it can provide before making a decision. Creating a supportive and comfortable home environment can significantly contribute to your overall well-being while living with arthritis.

Reducing Slips and Falls

Creating a slip-free environment in our homes is essential for ensuring safety. It begins with being mindful of the surfaces we walk on every day. For instance, rugs or mats can become hazards if they are not secured properly. Investing in non-slip pads or opting for rugs with rubber backing can make a significant difference. It's also wise to look closely at our flooring choices. Smooth surfaces like tiles or hardwood can sometimes be treacherous, especially when they get wet. Consider using anti-slip coatings on these surfaces to enhance safety.

Proper lighting is another key element in reducing slips and falls. Dimly lit areas can obscure potential hazards, making it difficult to navigate safely. Installing bright, energy-efficient bulbs and ensuring that each space is well-lit can lead to a dramatic decrease in accidents. Outdoor areas should also be considered. Keeping walkways clear of debris and ensuring handrails are installed in stairways is critical. As we strive to keep our families safe, having a designated place for shoes can prevent water and mud from spreading throughout the house, which may lead to slips.

The importance of textures and finishes in our homes cannot be overstated when it comes to enhancing grip. Using materials that have more texture can provide better footing, whether indoors or outdoors. For example, textured tiles in kitchens and bathrooms can significantly reduce the risk of slipping, especially when these areas are prone to moisture. When it comes to finishes—choosing paints that have a matte finish over glossy ones can also help. Glossy finishes are prone to reflect light, which can create glare and make it difficult to see any potential dangers lurking right in front of us. Adopting an awareness of these details can empower us to create safer spaces for ourselves and our loved ones. As we make these simple changes, let's remember that every small step leads to a giant leap toward safety.

By acknowledging the materials and methods we use in our homes, we can approach safety with empowerment rather than fear. Think about where you step each day and the surfaces underfoot. Investing in non-slip options doesn't just enhance safety; it promotes peace of mind for everyone who walks through your door. Take a few moments this week to assess your surroundings and make that small change—like placing a non-slip mat in your bathroom—because safety should never feel like a luxury. It's a priority we can all embrace.

Maintaining Clean and Safe Floors

Keeping our floors clean and clutter-free is essential for preventing accidents. I remember a time when I slipped on a stray toy left on the floor. It was a painful reminder of how clutter can lead to unexpected mishaps. The simple act of taking a few moments daily to tidy up can make a world of difference. Start by creating designated spots for frequently used items. When everything has its place, it becomes much easier to keep the floors clear. Encourage everyone in your household to participate in this routine. Together, you can transform your space into a safer environment for everyone.

Routine maintenance plays a crucial role in ensuring ongoing safety. Making cleaning a regular task can seem overwhelming at first, but breaking it down into manageable chunks can help. For instance, designating one day a week for a thorough cleaning is a great start. Each family member can be given specific duties, making the process more efficient and inclusive. This not only keeps the floors polished but also fosters teamwork. Additionally, consider investing in high-quality cleaning supplies that suit your floor type, whether it's hardwood, tile, or carpet. Better tools can lead to more effective cleaning results, making the entire process feel less daunting.

One practical tip to remember on this journey is to implement a no-shoe policy in your home. Shoes can carry dirt, grime, and even harmful chemicals. By inviting everyone to remove their shoes upon entering, you'll naturally reduce the amount of debris tracked into your space. Not only does this contribute to a cleaner floor, but it also helps create a more welcoming and hygienic home. By taking small, consistent steps, maintaining clean and safe floors can become an effortless part of your daily routine.

Softening Hard Surfaces

Walking on hard surfaces can be painful and exhausting, especially if you've spent hours on your feet. I've learned that incorporating soft surfaces into your living and working spaces can significantly cushion your feet and reduce impact. Consider the benefits of adding plush mats in areas where you stand for long periods, such as the kitchen or laundry room. These small changes make a noticeable difference in how your feet feel. Choosing materials like memory foam or gel cushioning is especially helpful as they adapt to your body, providing more support. Another option is to replace hard flooring with softer alternatives, like cork or bamboo. While they are naturally resilient, they also come with a bit of spring that feels great underfoot.   Adding softness doesn't stop at the floor. Some of my favorites are soft slippers or socks that provide a layer of cushioning as you move around your home. Even outdoor footwear that incorporates cushioning technology helps relieve pressure and is a fantastic way to keep your feet comfortable when you are on the go. Visualize stepping onto a surface that embraces your feet, instead of the hard ground that can zap your energy. It encourages you to keep exploring and enjoying your day fully.

When I decided to invest in area rugs and padded flooring, I experienced a transformation in my living space and my overall comfort. Area rugs can add a layer of softness that feels luxurious while also reducing noise. It's surprising how much a fluffy, inviting rug can warm up a room—not just in temperature but in atmosphere. The textures of rugs provide a gentle, cushioned feeling that invites you to kick off your shoes and get comfortable. You might find yourself spending more time lounging, reading, or engaging in activities that nurture your spirit. Padded flooring, on the other hand, offers a remarkable way to elevate not only the comfort of your feet but also your overall well-being. With cushioned surfaces, you could say goodbye to the aches and pains typically associated with walking on hard surfaces. It's a revelation to move about freely without the constant worry of discomfort. Additionally, with products specifically designed for impact absorption, you're likely to see the benefits during your fitness routines, whether you're doing yoga, dancing, or just exercising at home. Ultimately, whether it's through soft area rugs or supportive padded flooring, providing comfort in your environment enriches your journey, allowing you to tread softly wherever life takes you. Keeping a cozy rug or mat close by where you tend to spend the most time can serve as a gentle reminder to step lightly and prioritize comfort, nurturing not just your feet but your entire being.

Area Rugs: Safety and Style

When I first entered the world of interior design, I quickly learned that area rugs can serve as both a focal point and a safety feature in our homes. Choosing the right area rug goes beyond picking a color or pattern; it is essential to consider materials, textures, and placement to ensure safety. A well-chosen rug can provide comfort underfoot and help prevent slips and falls, especially in high-traffic areas or homes with young children and elderly residents. Opting for non-slip backings is a simple yet effective way to enhance safety, providing peace of mind while we walk through our spaces.

In addition to safety, the style of your area rug plays a significant role in enhancing your home's overall aesthetic. Rugs crafted from materials such as wool or synthetic fibers not only add a layer of coziness but also come in varying textures to suit your decor. The right rug can tie a room together, bringing harmony and warmth to your living spaces. Consider choosing a rug that complements the existing color palette and style of your home. This way, you can achieve both safety and beauty in a seamless manner.

Selecting an area rug that blends well with your home decor involves more than just matching colors. It starts with understanding the mood you want to create in each room. For example, a bright, bold rug can act as a statement piece in a neutral room, drawing attention and adding character. Conversely, if your space is already filled with vibrant colors and patterns, a more subtle, neutral rug can help ground the design, allowing other elements to shine.

Functionality is also an important aspect of design. Think about where the rug will be placed—under a dining table, in a living room, or in a bedroom—and how it will be used. A low-pile rug works well in a dining area, as it's easier to clean and won't trap crumbs as deeply as a high-pile option. Meanwhile, a plush rug in a bedroom can create a cozy retreat, enveloping your feet in softness as you step out of bed in the morning. Balance is key, and personal preferences should guide your choices.

Color is a powerful tool in design. Consider selecting rugs with tones that echo other features in your home, such as curtains or wall colors. This repetition creates a cohesive look that feels intentional and well thought out. Pay attention to the scale of patterns as well; large prints can open up a space visually, while smaller patterns can add details and texture. Always remember that your home should reflect your personality—select rugs that resonate with your soul while serving those functional purposes.

When you're ready to make a choice, take your time and don't rush the process. Exploring local stores or browsing online can provide inspiration. Many retailers even allow you to bring samples home, so you can see how they react with your wall colors and furnishings. Finally, giving thought to the rug maintenance will ensure its longevity, helping you appreciate both its beauty and functionality for years to come.

Chapter 5: Kitchen Modifications

Choosing the Right Kitchen Tools

When living with arthritis, even the simplest cooking tasks can feel daunting. Therefore, selecting ergonomic kitchen tools becomes crucial. Look for utensils with soft, padded grips that fit comfortably in your hand, allowing for a secure hold without straining your fingers. Consider pots and pans with wide handles that are easy to grasp and lightweight, making them manageable and reducing the risk of dropping them. Tools like can openers with built-in leverage or electric models can make opening jars and cans far less challenging. Invest in cutting boards that provide stability, preventing slipping while you chop. This way, you can enjoy the process of cooking without fighting against pain and discomfort.

Choosing tools that enhance comfort is a worthy investment for anyone, especially for those managing arthritis. Look into products designed specifically for ease of use, such as knives with larger, non-slip handles that require less force to operate. Many innovative kitchen gadgets are available today, from peelers to whisks, designed to minimize strain on your hands and wrists. It's also helpful to think about the layout of your kitchen. Organizing frequently used items within easy reach can eliminate unnecessary movements and make cooking feel more accessible. By prioritizing comfort and functionality, you will not only improve your cooking experience but also allow joy to return to the kitchen.

One practical tip that can transform your culinary experience is to use kitchen tools that adapt to different tasks. A simple device like a multi-functional food processor can take the place of several manual tools, significantly cutting down on the effort required for chopping, mixing, and blending. This reduces repetitive motion, which can aggravate joint pain. Remember, the right tools not only enhance your cooking but help create a more enjoyable and engaging experience in the kitchen.

Organizing Your Space for Efficiency

The kitchen can sometimes feel like a chaotic whirlwind when you're in the midst of preparing a meal. I've been there, flipping through drawers and rummaging through cabinets, only to find the spatula I need buried under a pile of unused utensils. Understanding how to organize your kitchen space can drastically change your experience, making the process smoother and more enjoyable. By grouping your tools and ingredients according to their logical use, you create a seamless flow that allows you to navigate with ease. For instance, keep all your cooking tools—like knives, cutting boards, and measuring cups—near the prep area. Similarly, place pots and pans close to the stove. Consider also designating a section of your counter for commonly used spices and oils, so they're just a reach away when you need them. When everything has its place, you not only save time but also reduce frustration, making cooking a much more relaxing and fulfilling experience.

Creating a workspace that promotes healthy movements is equally vital to maintaining your well-being while you cook. I've learned firsthand the importance of ergonomics in the kitchen. For example, when you're preparing food, standing on a surface that's too high can strain your back and legs. Try to ensure that your cutting boards and prep surfaces are at a comfortable height, ideally around waist level, to reduce bending and stretching. Also, consider investing in a good pair of shoes that offer support, allowing you to stand for longer periods without discomfort. As you work, take breaks to stretch your arms and legs. Shifting your weight from one foot to the other can also relieve tension.

Remember, cooking should be a joy, not a chore, and taking care of your body is part of that enjoyment.

Another practical tip to keep in mind is to declutter periodically. Regularly assessing what you use can free up space and ensure you're surrounded by the tools that serve you best. When everything is in its right place, both your spirit and productivity thrive. Set aside a little time to make adjustments in your kitchen and workspace; you'll find that even small changes can lead to a more efficient and pleasurable cooking experience.

Accessible Storage Solutions

Devising accessible storage methods can significantly ease the physical strain of everyday tasks and promote a more manageable living space. Instead of placing frequently used items in high cabinets or deep drawers, consider the benefits of lower shelving and pull-out drawers. These simple adjustments can minimize the need for bending or reaching, making life a little easier for everyone, especially those with mobility challenges. For instance, using clear bins on lower shelves can help you quickly spot what you need without the hassle of digging through stacks of containers. Organizing your items by use and frequency can transform your storage experience into one that supports your daily routines rather than hinders them.

Keeping frequently used items within easy reach is essential for maintaining an efficient and stress-free environment. When your most necessary tools and supplies are organized at a comfortable height, you save time and energy, making your day more productive. Think about the spaces you frequent the most—like your kitchen or bathroom. If you often reach for a particular spice or personal care item, prioritize placing them in dedicated, easily accessible locations. This could mean putting everyday spices in a categorized rack on the counter or moving essential toiletries from a high shelf to a rolling cart that sits at arm's length. Allowing yourself or those sharing your space the convenience of easy access will foster independence and increase confidence in managing daily tasks.

Consider a simple but effective tip: assess your frequently used items and evaluate their current placements. Are there adjustments that could make life easier, such as attaching hooks beside your door for keys and bags or using a tiered shelf in the pantry for easy visibility? Small changes can make a significant impact on your overall satisfaction and comfort in your environment.

Innovative Cooking Techniques

Cooking should be an enjoyable experience, but for many individuals with joint limitations, traditional methods can pose challenges. It is possible to explore adaptive cooking techniques that make the process more accessible and pleasurable. For instance, using tools with ergonomic handles can help minimize strain while chopping vegetables or stirring a pot. Investing in a good-quality food processor or blender can save time and energy, allowing you to create delicious meals without the need for intense manual work. Additionally, counter height can be adjusted with a simple platform that brings everything to your level, reducing the need to bend or stretch, which is important for those with arthritis or other joint issues. These alterations not only ensure your safety in the kitchen but also empower you to enjoy cooking, regardless of physical limitations.

Techniques that promote ease and comfort can significantly enhance your cooking experience. One effective method is employing slow cooking, which allows you to prepare meals with minimal effort. By placing ingredients in a slow cooker, you can enjoy flavorful, tender dishes without constant monitoring. Another helpful tip is to work in small, manageable increments. Preparing ingredients in advance, such as chopping vegetables or measuring spices, can make cooking feel less overwhelming and more inviting. Moreover, consider utilizing cooking utensils like automatic can openers or jar openers that require less grip strength. Each of these adjustments reduces the risk of pain and encourages a more enjoyable culinary journey.

Embracing innovations in cooking methods can truly transform your time in the kitchen. Small adjustments lead to big differences, ensuring that cooking remains a source of joy and creativity. Experimenting with these techniques not only enhances your culinary skills but also allows for a deeper connection with the food you prepare. Remember to listen to your body and adapt as needed, and don't hesitate to enlist the help of others when necessary. One practical tip is to keep your kitchen organized and stocked with the right tools, as accessing items easily can streamline the cooking process and keep your experience fun.

Adaptive Equipment for Meal Preparation

Adaptive equipment designed for meal preparation plays a crucial role in making cooking more accessible for individuals with disabilities or conditions that affect their ability to perform daily tasks. From cutting boards with stabilizing features to specially designed utensils that require less grip strength, these tools can transform the experience of cooking, making it not just feasible but enjoyable. When I first started using adaptive equipment, it was like a door opened up to a world where I could reclaim my independence in the kitchen. The sights and smells of food preparation, often overshadowed by frustrations, became a source of joy again. This transformation didn't happen overnight, but each small tool introduced into my routine made a significant impact on my ability to participate in meal prep with confidence and creativity.

The benefits of using innovative tools for enhancing independence are remarkable. For many, cooking is not just about nourishment; it's a form of self-expression and a way to connect with loved ones. Using adaptive equipment can boost self-esteem and foster a sense of pride as individuals prepare meals that are enjoyed by family and friends. I recall the first dinner I made entirely on my own using adaptive gadgets; the joy on my family's faces was priceless. Innovations like ergonomic peelers or easy-grip knives allow individuals to engage more effectively, ensuring that meal preparation is not just an obligation but a delightful activity. These tools not only enable independence but also support social interaction and communication during meal times, giving people the chance to share experiences and create lasting memories in the kitchen.

When embracing adaptive equipment, it's important to explore different options to find what works best for your unique needs. Often, local organizations or online communities offer demonstrations or resources to help individuals find the right tools. Don't hesitate to reach out and ask for support; you're not alone in this journey. A practical tip I learned through experience is to start with a few essential items that cater to your most pressing challenges in the kitchen. Gradually introducing new tools, rather than feeling overwhelmed by a full set of options all at once, can lead to a more comfortable and enjoyable adaptation process. The kitchen can be a place of creativity and connection, and with the right adaptive equipment, it becomes a space where everyone can thrive.

Chapter 6: Bathroom Adjustments

Walk-in Showers vs. Bathtubs

When considering the differences between walk-in showers and bathtubs, accessibility and safety become paramount, especially for those of us navigating the challenges that can come with aging or physical limitations. Walk-in showers often provide a seamless entry designed to reduce the risk of slips and falls, which is a crucial factor for many. They typically feature non-slip flooring, grab bars, and a low or no threshold, allowing individuals to step in and out with ease. On the other hand, traditional bathtubs may present some challenges. Getting in and out of a tub can require a bit of agility, and for someone with mobility concerns, this can easily turn into a risky endeavor. However, many people find comfort in a bathtub's warmth and soothing waters, which can offer a sense of relaxation that's hard to replicate in a shower. The choice often comes down to individual circumstances and preferences, which we'll explore further.

Reflecting on your own situation can help guide you toward the option that feels right for you. Assess your bath time rituals and what you truly enjoy. Do you see bathing as a moment of relaxation, a luxurious escape after a long day? Perhaps a bathtub is your haven. Or maybe efficiency and safety in your routine are your top priorities. In that case, a walk-in shower may serve you better. Think about how each option fits within your personal lifestyle and needs. Imagine stepping into a warm, inviting bath or the refreshing burst of water in a quick shower. Whatever resonates with you matters. Embrace your preferences and don't hesitate to talk to family members or professionals who can offer insights based on experiences similar to yours. This personal assessment isn't just about plumbing fixtures; it's about your comfort, well-being, and safety.

It's essential to consider both the functional aspects and the emotional connections we have with bathing. Sometimes, we underestimate the profound impact that our bathing experience can have on our mood and daily routine. Whichever option you lean towards, don't forget to think about customizable features, such as shower benches or more supportive tub styles, that can make your choice even more accommodating. Having a well-thought-out bathroom setup can significantly enhance your sense of independence and ease. Take a moment to envision what would make your bathing experience delightful, whether it's the freedom of a walk-in shower or the tranquil retreat of a bathtub. This moment of reflection could lead you to a decision that transforms your personal space.

Grab Bars and Handheld Showers

Installing grab bars in the bathroom can make a significant difference in safety and independence. For many people, especially those with mobility issues, the bathroom can feel like a risky place. Standing on slippery tiles and navigating the tub or shower can be daunting. Having grab bars installed can provide that extra layer of support. They act like a reassuring hand, ready to assist whenever it's needed. Whenever I step into my bathroom, I feel a wave of relief knowing I have something sturdy to hold onto. The reassurance that comes with knowing I can safely lean or pull myself up is invaluable. Grab bars can be discreet, blending in with your bathroom's decor while serving the crucial function of preventing falls. They not only enhance safety but also foster a sense of confidence, allowing individuals to maintain their independence. Being able to bathe without fear of falling or losing balance transforms a potentially stressful routine into a calming experience.

Handheld showers significantly improve the bathing experience by providing convenience and flexibility. Unlike traditional fixed showerheads, handheld options can be adjusted to suit personal preferences. They allow the user full control over where the water flows, making it easier to clean oneself, especially for those with limited mobility. Just the thought of being able to sit comfortably on a shower chair and easily reach the showerhead brings a sense of peace. It becomes a pleasant experience rather than a chore. With a handheld shower, I can direct the water exactly where I need it, eliminating awkward maneuvers that often lead to discomfort or frustration. This simple tool empowers individuals to maintain personal hygiene without assistance, preserving dignity and privacy. Beyond just practicality, handheld showers can also transform bathing from a routine task into a soothing experience that promotes relaxation and well-being. The gentle flow of water and the freedom to adjust it to my liking have turned shower time into a ritual of self-care.

Combining grab bars with a handheld shower can create an incredibly supportive and functional bathroom environment. Together, they cater to the unique needs of individuals who may struggle with balance or mobility. By enhancing safety and ease of use, they foster a greater sense of security and autonomy in daily routines. It's worth noting that investing in such modifications is not merely about addressing current challenges; it's about paving the way for a more comfortable future. Taking the step to install these features is a powerful decision towards greater independence and improved quality of life. For anyone contemplating these changes, it's often helpful to consult with a professional to ensure the right placements and styles are selected for optimal safety and comfort.

Non-slip Mats and Flooring

When it comes to enhancing safety in the bathroom, choosing the right non-slip mats and flooring is essential. Look for mats made from high-quality rubber or textured materials that naturally resist slipping. These materials provide a robust grip underfoot, especially when wet. Additionally, consider the thickness of the mat; thicker, more substantial mats often offer better cushioning and stability, reducing the risk of slips. Pay attention to the edges of the mats as well. A design with straight or beveled edges reduces the likelihood of tripping while entering or exiting the shower or tub. Lastly, it's critical to ensure that the mats can be easily cleaned and are resistant to mold and mildew, keeping your bathroom hygienic and safe.

The role of traction in preventing falls cannot be overstated. The surface texture of non-slip flooring plays a pivotal role in providing the grip you need, especially in moist environments like the bathroom. The more traction you have, the less chance there is for a slip to occur. In my experience, choosing flooring with a coarse surface, rather than glossy tiles, can significantly reduce the risk of accidents. Let's not forget that all the prevention measures mean little if they aren't regularly maintained. Regularly check mats and flooring for wear and tear, replacing them when necessary to ensure that they continue to provide safe surfaces to walk on. Each step taken should bring confidence rather than uncertainty.

To enhance the effectiveness of your non-slip solutions, consider layering them, such as placing non-slip mats over existing flooring or using additional textured bath mats. Creating a cohesive safety plan in the bathroom involves not only choosing the right materials but also ensuring that they work well together. Surround yourself with supportive, safe environments that foster confidence and reduce the risk of falls. Your bathroom should be a place of relaxation, not worry, so taking proactive steps to enhance its safety will lead to a more enjoyable experience.

Accessible Sink and Vanity Design

Designing sinks and vanities with accessibility in mind transforms daily routines into effortless experiences. The height at which sinks are installed is crucial. When considering the best height, it's important to keep in mind the varying needs of individuals, especially those who might be seated while performing personal care tasks. Ideally, a sink should be between 28 and 34 inches from the floor, which accommodates both standing and seated users. Additionally, ensuring that the sink has an open space beneath can enhance accessibility, allowing for wheelchairs and other mobility aids to fit comfortably underneath. The reach to faucets and soap dispensers is also vital. Lever-style handles or touchless sensors can make getting water easier for everyone, allowing for a simple push or tap rather than a complicated twist that requires grip strength.

Making personal care routines easier to manage can significantly enhance the quality of life. Simple additions can make a world of difference, such as a wall-mounted mirror that tilts and adjusts for better visibility from different angles. Consider also implementing lower shelves or accessible storage solutions in the vanity. Pull-out drawers that slide out easily can help keep essentials within reach, reducing the need for bending or stretching. This organization promotes independence, making it less daunting to access grooming tools or hygiene products. Additionally, incorporating grab bars near the sink can provide extra support and stability while moving around, ensuring safety is a priority without sacrificing style.

One practical tip is to think about the materials used for sinks and vanities. Smooth surfaces that are easy to clean and maintain, along with non-slip flooring, can make the bathroom safer and more user-friendly. Soft lighting around the vanity not only enhances visibility but also creates a welcoming environment. Elevating the comfort and accessibility of these spaces is a journey worth taking, and every small adjustment contributes to a more inclusive and supportive environment.

Lighting for Visibility and Safety

Ensuring that the bathroom is well-lit is essential for reducing conflict, both physically and emotionally. Adequate lighting can make a significant difference in how we navigate this space, particularly in a room often filled with hard surfaces and potential hazards. I remember a time when I nearly slipped on a wet floor simply because the lighting was dim, and shadows concealed the dangers awaiting underfoot. By incorporating bright, even lighting fixtures, we can illuminate every corner, minimize shadows, and create an environment where movement feels safe and secure. For those who may struggle with mobility, such as seniors or individuals recovering from injury, lighting becomes even more crucial. Simple changes, such as adding brighter bulbs or strategically placing light sources near pathways, can transform a once hazardous room into a welcoming oasis of comfort and safety.

Proper lighting doesn't just enhance visibility; it can also uplift our spirits and boost confidence. When we can see clearly, we are more likely to take our time, appreciate our reflections, and engage in self-care routines without fear or hesitation. In my own experience, I have found that having well-placed lights around mirrors and counters helps me feel empowered rather than rushed or anxious. Illuminate those areas well, and you create an atmosphere where one can truly take a moment to breathe and appreciate themselves. Good lighting fosters a sense of control and encourages positive body image, which, in turn, enhances overall safety—both emotional and physical. This is particularly important in a space like the bathroom, where the subtle act of grooming can greatly influence how we carry ourselves throughout the day.

As you think about enhancing your bathroom lighting, consider incorporating layers of light. Combining ambient lighting with task lighting creates a dynamic environment that not only serves practical needs but also promotes a soothing atmosphere. A soft overhead light might create a calming backdrop, while bright fixtures around the mirror provide the clarity needed for those close-up tasks like shaving or applying makeup. This thoughtful approach can transform even the simplest routines into a nurturing experience, reminding us that safety and self-care can go hand in hand. By taking these small yet impactful steps, you open the door to a more confident, comfortable, and safe experience every time you step into your bathroom.

Chapter 7: Living Room Comfort

Choosing the Right Seating

Selecting comfortable seating options is crucial for maintaining joint health. I once overlooked this aspect, thinking any chair was good enough. But as I adapted to a more active lifestyle, I learned that the right seating could support my body in ways I never imagined. It's essential to consider chairs that allow your spine to maintain its natural curve. Look for options that come with adequate lumbar support, which alleviates stress on your lower back. When sitting, your feet should rest flat on the ground with your knees at a 90-degree angle. If your chair doesn't support this position, it could lead to stiffness and pain, especially if you spend long hours sitting. Memory foam cushions or ergonomic chairs can make a significant difference. They contour to your body, distributing your weight evenly and reducing pressure on your joints.

The importance of proper support for relaxation and comfort cannot be overstated. After spending countless hours on poorly supportive furniture, I found myself fatigued and unable to enjoy moments of rest. A good chair should not only provide physical support but should also invite you to relax. Consider seating that encourages good posture while being plush enough to sink into. Look for recliners or lounge chairs with adjustable features, so you can customize your position depending on your mood or activity. When you settle into a chair that feels good, you can unwind and leave the stress of the day behind. Your body deserves that little haven of comfort. Always remember that investing in the right seating is investing in your overall well-being. Make it a priority to seek out chairs that resonate with your needs and preferences. Comfort is not just a luxury; it's a necessity for a healthy, fulfilling life.

A practical tip to ensure your seating supports joint health is to take the time to test a chair before making a purchase. Spend a few moments sitting in different positions to see how it feels. If you feel any discomfort shortly after sitting down, it's a good indication that the chair may not be the right fit. Prioritize your comfort, and don't hesitate to ask for guidance from sales associates who are trained in ergonomic design. Remember, a little diligence in finding the right seating can lead to years of comfort and support, enhancing your quality of life significantly.

Accessorizing for Accessibility

Transforming a living space into a more accessible environment can be as simple as thoughtfully selecting the right accessories. Imagine how a beautiful, brightly colored rug can not only tie a room together aesthetically but also provide traction for stability, making it safer to navigate. An eye-catching lamp with an easy-to-reach switch can illuminate your favorite reading corner while ensuring you don't have to strain to turn it on or off. Consider using multi-functional furniture, such as an ottoman that doubles as storage. This way, you keep your space organized and can easily access items without rummaging around. Adding hooks or wall-mounted baskets can also clear up floor space and make everyday items more readily available, encapsulating the perfect blend of style and utility.

The right accessories can elevate a space not just in functionality but also in how it feels. Think about a stylish adaptive handle for your kitchen cabinets that aligns with your design aesthetics while providing ease of grip and use. It's amazing how something as simple as color can impact our mood. Vibrant, uplifting hues can breathe life into a room and make tasks feel less daunting. For instance, a cheerful, patterned shower curtain can brighten your bathroom, making it a more welcoming space. Integrating artistic elements like sculptures or wall art, placed at the right accessibility height, adds layers of personality to your environment while ensuring that each piece is within reach. The blend of function and style is not just about meeting your needs; it's about creating an environment where you can thrive.

Creating Space for Movement

Arranging furniture in a way that promotes easy movement can transform your living space into an inviting environment. Begin by envisioning how you use your space. Consider pathways; they should flow naturally and be easily navigated without any obstacles. It's important to avoid heavy, bulky furniture that restricts movement. Instead, opt for lighter pieces that can be easily rearranged depending on your needs. Positioning larger furniture, like sofas and chairs, away from high-traffic areas creates open paths. Make use of multi-functional furniture; for example, a coffee table that doubles as storage can free up additional space while providing practical functionality.

Creating an environment that encourages active living goes hand in hand with the layout of your home. You want your living space not just to look good, but to actively inspire movement. Consider incorporating designated activity zones, even in limited spaces. A corner of a room could be transformed into a small workout area with a yoga mat and a few weights. Doing so invites a sense of purpose to that space. Additionally, choose decorative elements that align with a vibrant lifestyle, such as artwork that reflects outdoor scenes or motivational quotes about movement and health. These elements can provoke thoughts of activity and invigorate your day.

To further enhance the ambiance, open up your space to natural light and fresh air. This connection to nature not only brightens your home but also uplifts your spirit, prompting a more active lifestyle. Every small change contributes to a larger shift towards wellness. Start with one area of your home and make it a space that invites movement, allows you to breathe freely, and compels you to embrace each day with enthusiasm. If you want to take a practical step today, start by rearranging just one room; it might spark new routines and invigorate your daily life.

Lighting Considerations

Natural and artificial lighting play a crucial role in our lives, affecting both safety and ambiance. Consider the way light streams into your home from windows during the day. It brings warmth, creates a sense of space, and even influences our mood. When I first moved into my home, I often found myself feeling slightly disoriented in dimly lit rooms. It wasn't until I began to recognize the importance of good lighting that I realized how it can deeply impact our well-being. Proper lighting can help prevent accidents, making it easier to navigate spaces without stumbling, while also fostering a positive emotional environment that invites creativity and relaxation. Without adequate light, a room can feel oppressive, and we can miss out on the joy that sunlight brings, not to mention the added magic of evening settings enhanced by thoughtfully placed lamps and fixtures.

To optimize lighting conditions in the living room, it's helpful to be intentional with your setup. Begin by assessing where natural light enters your space. Large windows are a blessing, but if your living room lacks direct sunlight, consider using mirrors to reflect light and brighten up corners. Layering light sources is another effective strategy; combining ambient, task, and accent lighting can transform your living room into a welcoming haven. For example, use a soft overhead fixture paired with stylish table lamps to create a cozy atmosphere in the evening hours. These layers help to eliminate harsh shadows and provide flexibility to change the mood based on the time of day or occasion. You can even experiment with dimmer switches, allowing you to adjust the brightness according to your needs, whether it's a lively gathering or a quiet night with a book.

Investing in lightbulbs that mimic natural daylight can further enhance your space. These bulbs are not only energy-efficient but can invigorate a room, making it feel fresh and lively. Moreover, incorporating smart lighting solutions can help you control the ambiance with a simple app or voice command, tailoring your environment to match your feelings. By focusing on these lighting considerations, you can create a nurturing space that feels safe, inviting, and alive—a true reflection of your personality and lifestyle.

Ergonomic Entertainment Systems

Setting up an entertainment system that prioritizes ease of use can transform your experience from frustrating to enjoyable. When bringing together various components—like a television, sound system, and gaming console—consider how you interact with each device. Position your TV at eye level to avoid straining your neck and ensure that the seating is at a comfortable distance. The layout should encourage relaxation rather than forcing you to stretch or twist your body unnaturally. Using a universal remote or smart home integration can simplify your interactions, allowing you to control everything from lighting to volume with a single click. Think about your media storage as well; keeping everything organized can help reduce clutter and distractions, allowing you to focus on what matters: enjoying your favorite shows, movies, or games.

Incorporating technology that enhances comfort can elevate your leisure time significantly. Adjustable seating with built-in support can encourage better posture while allowing you to sink into relaxation. Consider furniture with features like recline and lumbar support, perfect for those binge-watching sessions or long gaming nights. Sound systems that offer surround sound can provide an immersive experience, transporting you into the action without the discomfort of bad acoustics. Smart lighting solutions that automatically adjust not only create the perfect ambiance but also help reduce eye strain after extended viewing periods. Don't underestimate the power of blankets and cushions—having materials that feel good against your skin can turn a regular evening into a cozy escape.

Creating an ergonomic entertainment setup is about more than just comfort; it's also about how these choices impact your overall well-being. Investing in a quality chair or couch, for instance, not only enhances your entertainment experience but also contributes to your health. The right technology and furniture can encourage you to engage in leisure activities without the wear and tear that often comes with poor ergonomics. To get the most from your entertainment experiences, take a moment to evaluate your system and make adjustments where necessary. Incorporate elements that cater to your comfort and enjoyment— those small changes can lead to a more enriching leisure time you truly deserve.

Chapter 8: Bedroom Enhancements

Choosing the Best Mattress

When it comes to selecting a mattress, the right support is crucial for achieving restful sleep. After experiencing many sleepless nights on the wrong mattress, I learned that comfort is more than just a fluffy surface. It's about alignment and support for your body. Your mattress should keep your spine aligned, relieving pressure from areas where tension can build, such as your shoulders, hips, and lower back. Think about your sleeping position as you explore options; side sleepers often need a softer feel to cushion the shoulders, while back or stomach sleepers might require a firmer base to keep their spine supported. Don't overlook your weight and body type either, as these factors affect how a mattress feels under you. A heavier person may sink more into a softer mattress and miss out on the necessary support, while lighter individuals might find firmer options uncomfortable. Therefore, a careful evaluation of your unique body needs will lead you to the right mattress choice, promoting better sleep hygiene that enhances your daily life.

The importance of testing different options cannot be overstated when it comes to finding your ideal mattress. It's easy to get caught up in brands and marketing claims, but nothing beats the experience of lying down on a mattress and giving it a real test run. This is your moment to see how it fits you, literally. I remember stepping into a showroom feeling overwhelmed by the choices. However, once I started to explore, moving from bed to bed, I felt the physical differences. For me, the key was taking my time. Lie down in your natural sleeping position for at least ten minutes. Pay attention to how it feels under your body and how well it supports your spine. Bring your partner along if you share your bed; different preferences are common, so consideration of both people's needs is essential. Engage in the process and trust your instincts as you navigate this decision. It's an investment in your well-being, and you deserve to choose the mattress that makes you wake up feeling refreshed and ready for whatever lies ahead.

When entering the world of mattresses, remember to keep an open mind and prioritize comfort. Allow yourself to explore various materials—from memory foam to innerspring and hybrid options. Each has its unique benefits, and understanding what resonates with you will aid in narrowing down your choices. Take advantage of trial periods many companies offer since this can basically be a risk-free opportunity to confirm that your choice is right for your sleep style. Most importantly, don't rush the process. Sleep impacts every part of your life, and investing time in selecting the perfect mattress ensures that your nights are restorative and your days are rejuvenated.

Bedding and Sleep Comfort

Creating a serene sleep environment begins with selecting the right bedding materials. The feel of the fabric against your skin can greatly influence how well you rest each night. Natural fibers like cotton, linen, and bamboo are excellent choices because they allow your skin to breathe and maintain a comfortable temperature. Cotton, for instance, is soft and absorbent, making it ideal for a cozy bed. Linen, made from flax, provides a unique texture that not only looks beautiful but also offers incredible durability and a lovely, relaxed feel as it softens over time. Bamboo has gained popularity for its natural hypoallergenic properties while also being moisture-wicking. Think about the climate you live in; if it's humid, opt for breathable materials that help you stay cool.

If you suffer from allergies or have sensitive skin, hypoallergenic bedding is a fantastic option that ensures you feel comfortable while you sleep. Materials such as polyester or specific cotton blends are designed to resist allergens like dust mites and mold. They provide a sense of relief and comfort that encourages better sleep without worrying about irritants. Additionally, consider investing in organic bedding. Organic cotton, produced without harmful chemicals, is gentler on your skin and the environment. Discovering materials that work for you personally can lead to a more restful night. Don't underestimate the power of a good pillow and mattress; selecting ones with hypoallergenic properties can dramatically enhance your sleeping experience.

Remember to prioritize comfort when choosing bedding, allowing yourself the luxury of investing in quality materials. This not only enhances your sleep but positively impacts your wellbeing overall. As you explore different options, take the time to feel the textures and understand what will make your sleep environment a nurturing refuge. Before making a purchase, always read labels and opt for certified materials that align with your needs, creating a space that supports restful, rejuvenating sleep.

Mobility Aids for Getting In and Out of Bed

When it comes to getting in and out of bed, having the right mobility aids can make all the difference in maintaining independence and ensuring safety. Devices such as bed rails offer a sturdy grip that can help you lift yourself into a sitting position or support you as you stand. These rails come in various styles, some that attach to the bed frame while others are designed to be portable, making it easier to transfer them from one bed to another. Another excellent option is a transfer pole, which can be installed near your bed. With a strong vertical support, it helps you pivot and maneuver when transitioning from lying down to standing up. Consider also a bedside commode; while it aids with bathroom visits, it also allows you to remain close to your bed. And, if mobility is a concern, a bed wedge or adjustable bed base can help elevate the head of the bed for easier access and comfort, allowing you to slide more effortlessly into a seated position.

Beyond mechanical aids, creating a safe environment around your bed can greatly enhance your overall experience. Simple changes, like keeping essential items within reach—like your phone, glasses, or water—can minimize the need to stretch or strain. Non-slip mats near the bed can help prevent falls. Adequate lighting is essential too; having a bedside lamp or night light ensures you can see where you're going when the room is dark. If possible, involve family or caregivers in discussing these solutions, as their support can empower your journey to greater independence. Remember, even the smallest adaptations can significantly impact your safety and comfort. It's about equipping yourself with the tools and knowledge needed to reclaim your space and autonomy, making daily routines feel more manageable and less intimidating.

One practical tip is to practice the movements you need to make from your bed during the day, when you feel more energetic. This way, you can build confidence in your abilities, refine your techniques, and discover the right aids that suit your needs best. Take it slow, and remember that every effort counts towards living more boldly and independently.

Decluttering for Peace of Mind

Living in a cluttered environment can weigh heavily on the mind. When I finally decided to declutter my bedroom, I felt an instant lift in my mental clarity. A clutter-free space is not just about aesthetics; it significantly contributes to reducing stress. Every item in your room holds a piece of energy. When surrounded by unnecessary items, your mind can become preoccupied with thoughts of chaos and disorder. It's easy to become overwhelmed, and I found that once my bedroom was organized and free of distractions, I could think more clearly. With a neat space, my focus sharpened, and I was far less anxious. The simplicity and tranquility I created in my bedroom mirrored the internal peace I craved.

To enhance your sleep environment, consider a few strategic decluttering tips. Start by removing anything that doesn't serve a purpose in your bedroom. I began with everything from old clothes to sentimental items that no longer brought me joy. You might be surprised to find how many things collect dust, not adding value to your life. Next, think about the colors and materials around you. Ideally, your sleep surroundings should be calming. Opt for soothing colors and keep your decor minimal. Creating a space dedicated solely to rest can amplify your sleep quality. I also encourage you to create a nighttime ritual, which can include spending those last moments of the day setting aside items or tasks for the next day. This practice not only clears your space but also clears your mind, making room for restorative sleep.

Remember, decluttering is not a one-time task but a continuous process. Regularly reassess your belongings and keep an eye on the energy in your space. A practical tip: create a small 'donate' box that you can easily access. Whenever you find something that you no longer need, toss it in the box. This small action maintains your decluttered space and assists in creating a habit of letting go, making your quest for peace of mind much more attainable.

Creating a Relaxed Sleep Environment

Transforming your bedroom into a calm and soothing sanctuary starts with careful attention to how you set up the space. Begin by decluttering the room, as a tidy environment helps to ease the mind and invites relaxation. Consider using soft, neutral colors for your walls and decor, as these hues evoke a sense of tranquility. Choosing the right bedding is crucial; opt for high-quality, breathable fabrics that feel gentle against your skin. Creating a cozy nook with plush pillows and a weighted blanket can add an extra layer of comfort. Keep the bedroom dark and cool, as a lower temperature can help signal your body that it's time to sleep. Finally, think about the layout of your furniture. Arrange your bed so it feels inviting and not obstructed, making it the focal point of the room. This deliberate setup can help to establish a relaxing mindset as you enter your personal retreat each night.

Incorporating sensory elements can significantly enhance your sleep environment. Soft, ambient sounds can create a serene atmosphere; consider using a white noise machine or playing gentle music that lulls you into relaxation. Natural sounds, like ocean waves or a gentle rain, might also be soothing and aid in sleep onset. Light plays an equally important role. Invest in blackout curtains to block disruptive streetlights and allow for a deep, restful sleep. Alternatively, use dimmable lights or bedside lamps with warm bulbs to create a soft glow as you wind down in the evening. This gradual dimming can signal to your brain that it's time to relax. Additionally, introducing aromatic elements can enhance your sleep experience; essential oils like lavender or chamomile have calming properties. Consider using a diffuser or simply placing a few drops of oil on your pillow to immerse yourself in their soothing scents as you drift off.

Remember that creating a sleep sanctuary is a personal endeavor. Experiment with different elements until you discover what makes you feel most at peace. Tailoring your sleep environment to your preferences can not only enhance your ability to fall asleep but also improve the quality of your rest. Make small adjustments over time, and soon enough, you will find your own unique blend of comfort that leads to rejuvenating night after night.

Chapter 9: Home Office Adaptations

Setting Up an Ergonomic Workspace

Creating an ergonomic workspace is a vital step toward maintaining joint health and overall well-being. It begins with the fundamental elements that should be present in your work environment. A good chair is the cornerstone. It should provide adequate lumbar support, allowing your lower back to rest comfortably while maintaining the natural curve of your spine. Choose a chair that allows your feet to rest flat on the floor or on a footrest, with your knees at or slightly below the level of your hips, which helps in preventing strain on your joints.

Your desk height is equally important. Ideally, your workspace should be at a level that allows your elbows to rest comfortably at a 90-degree angle while typing. This simple adjustment can do wonders for our shoulders and wrists, minimizing the risk of developing pain over time. Consider adding a detachable keyboard and mouse if your desk is too high or low, making it easier to find that perfect position.

The placement of your monitor plays a significant role as well. Eyes should be at the same level as the top of the screen, allowing you to look slightly downward when viewing the middle of the monitor. This positioning helps to maintain a neutral neck position and reduces strain, enhancing your comfort while working long hours. Good lighting is also essential; it not only prevents eye strain but can also affect your overall mood and productivity.

Posture is often overlooked, but it can greatly influence how we feel during our workday. When sitting, align your body so that your head is stacked over your spine, your shoulders are relaxed, and your elbows remain close to your body. This position can help avoid discomfort and potential injury. It might take time to develop a more mindful approach to sitting correctly, but the initial discomfort you may feel as you adjust is a small price to pay for a healthier posture.

Incorporating short breaks into your work routine can also serve as a powerful tool for improving posture. Stand up, stretch, and walk for a few minutes every hour. These simple movements combat the stiffness that can accumulate from prolonged sitting. Taking moments to realign your body will promote blood flow and increase your energy, making it easier to return to your tasks with renewed focus.

Choosing the Right Office Chair

An ideal office chair is more than just a place to sit; it's an investment in your health and productivity. When it comes to comfort, look for a chair with adjustable features that can cater to your specific needs. A chair that allows you to modify the height, lumbar support, and armrests can significantly reduce strain during those long hours of work. I've learned that a well-designed chair promotes good posture by providing adequate support to your back, which helps to prevent fatigue and discomfort. Opt for a design that has breathable fabric or mesh as this will keep you cool and comfortable even on the busiest days. The right chair should fit your body perfectly, cradling you in support without being overly rigid. Your chair should allow you to easily shift your position throughout the day, keeping your body engaged and your mind alert.

Investing in quality seating that suits your body type is crucial. I remember when I first realized the impact my office chair had on my overall well-being. I decided to spend a little more money on a chair tailored to my frame, and it changed everything. Not only did I feel more comfortable, but my productivity skyrocketed as well. It's easy to overlook the importance of a chair when you're starting out or trying to save costs, but a good chair is a game changer. Prioritize your body and don't settle for discomfort. Everyone's physique is unique, and there's no one-size-fits-all solution. So, take the time to find a chair that feels right for you, one that allows you to work without the dreaded aches and pains that come from poor support. Remember, investing in your comfort is investing in your success.

Before you make a decision, consider trying out different chairs to see which one feels best. Some stores allow test sitting, giving you a chance to feel the fit and support before purchasing. This thoughtful step could save you from discomfort in the future. Trust your instincts; if a chair feels right, it probably is. Also, as you assess your choices, remember to think about the long-term benefits. A good chair might seem like an expense now, but it can prevent health issues down the line, making it a worthwhile investment for your comfort and productivity.

Desk Arrangement for Comfort

Setting up your desk for maximum ease and accessibility requires thoughtful consideration of how you use your space. Imagine sitting comfortably at your desk, ready to dive into your work. The first step is to assess your chair and desk height. Your chair should allow your feet to rest flat on the floor with your knees at a right angle. If your desk is too high or too low, it can lead to discomfort and strain over time. Adjusting the height of your chair or desk can make all the difference. If you're on the shorter side, consider using a footrest to maintain that ergonomic position that keeps you comfortable for long periods of work.

Your computer screen should be positioned at eye level to reduce neck strain. This means placing your monitor an arm's length away, at a height where your eye naturally rests on the top third of the screen. If you type a lot, ensuring that your keyboard is at a comfortable height is crucial. Your wrists should be straight as you type, possibly using a wrist pad for extra support. Having your mouse nearby and within the same plane as your keyboard will help minimize the awkward stretching that can lead to discomfort.

Once you have the essentials arranged, focus on keeping everything you need within arm's reach. This includes your notebook, pens, and any other materials you frequently utilize. By organizing your workspace with drawer dividers or desktop organizers, you minimize clutter and can find what you need quickly. A tidy workspace reduces stress and distraction. Consider using a small caddy for often-used items, so you can easily push it aside when you need more space, keeping your area adaptable to your immediate needs. Make it a habit to tidy your desk at the end of each day. It ensures that you return to a clean, inviting space that motivates you to get back to work with enthusiasm.

A practical tip to enhance comfort is to incorporate small breaks into your routine. Stand, stretch, and move around every hour, which not only helps with circulation but can invigorate your focus. Remember, a well-organized, comfortable desk can dramatically impact your productivity and overall well-being.

Technology Tools for Accessibility

Living with arthritis can deeply impact everyday tasks, especially when it comes to using technology. Many devices and programs are designed with accessibility in mind, aiming to ease the stress on our joints and make interactions more manageable. Voice recognition software allows users to control their computers and send messages without needing to type, creating a more comfortable experience. Touchscreen devices often provide larger buttons and different sensitivity settings, making it easier for those with limited dexterity to navigate. Adaptive tools, like styluses designed for ease of grip, can also help alleviate the strain caused by traditional writing utensils. Overall, the goal of these technologies is to provide support and enable smoother communication, so that we can continue engaging with the world without added discomfort.

For day-to-day computer tasks, several tools can significantly enhance your experience. For instance, ergonomic keyboards and mice are specifically designed to promote a natural hand position, reducing the strain on fingers and wrists. Many models offer comfortable grips and customizable buttons that allow for easier functionality. Voice-controlled applications, such as dictation tools, can transform how we interact with text, helping to eliminate the repetitive motion of typing. Additionally, screen readers are invaluable for those with visual impairments linked to arthritic conditions; they provide audio feedback, making navigation simple and effective. Assistive technology can seem daunting at first, yet it is welcoming and supportive, ready to assist you in managing your workflow with ease.

Finding the right tools often involves a bit of trial and error. It's important to remember that each piece of technology can be pivotal in reclaiming control over daily tasks. Adapting to new devices takes time, but the rewards are worth it—think improved comfort, efficiency, and ultimately, a more fulfilling day-to-day life. Whenever you're exploring new technology, consider starting with tools that resonate with your personal needs. Design choices that offer unique ergonomics and user interfaces can transform how you experience working or engaging with others online. A focused approach to selecting your tools can lead to surprising improvements in your daily routine.

Promoting Movement Throughout the Day

Incorporating movement into your workday is crucial for combating the stiffness and pain that often accompany prolonged sitting. Many of us experience discomfort in our bodies as we navigate through tasks and meetings, often forgetting how vital it is to stay active. I've been there myself—sitting at my desk for hours, lost in work, and feeling the creaks and aches set in. It's a silent struggle that many face, and it's easy to clamp down on those sensations, assuming they're just part of the daily grind. However, I've come to understand that prioritizing movement doesn't just alleviate discomfort; it enhances overall well-being and productivity.

Finding ways to stretch and move throughout your day doesn't require a lot of time or space. Simple stretches can be performed right at your desk, seamlessly integrating into your routine. For instance, while sitting, try rolling your shoulders back and forth, letting the tension melt away with each rotation. You can also keep your feet flat on the ground and, one at a time, lift your toes, flexing your feet to ease tightness in the calves. When you feel comfortable, stand up and reach your arms overhead, stretching toward the ceiling as if trying to grab a cloud. This movement not only opens up your chest but also energizes your mind. Even a simple neck stretch can do wonders—gently tilting your head from side to side can release built-up stress and encourage better blood flow to your brain.

Incorporating these small movements, even just for a few minutes every hour, can create a big impact.

Perhaps set a timer as a reminder to stand, stretch, and take deep breaths. The key is consistency; making it a habit will foster a sense of rejuvenation and focus. Remember, the intent is not about strenuous exercise; it's about embracing gentle movements that allow your body to feel alive, refreshed, and fully engaged throughout the day. So, as you navigate your tasks, consider creating a personal routine of movements that resonate with you, and allow your body to express gratitude for the simple act of movement.

Chapter 10: Outdoor Accessibility

Gardening for Arthritis Care

Gardening can be a wonderful source of relief for those living with arthritis. It offers a unique blend of physical activity and mindfulness that can truly help ease symptoms. When you dig your hands into the soil, there's something incredibly grounding and soothing about the simple act of nurturing a plant. This connection to nature is not just refreshing; it's therapeutic. Many who suffer from arthritis find that tending to their garden allows them to experience a sense of accomplishment and joy. It can lift your spirits and provide a welcome distraction from the daily pain that often accompanies the condition.

Additionally, being outside in the fresh air and sunlight benefits your overall mood and can even lessen feelings of isolation that often accompany chronic illnesses. Watching a seed grow into a plant can be a metaphor for hope and resilience, inspiring you to embrace your own journey with arthritis. The rhythmic motions of planting seeds, watering, and pruning can also serve as light exercise. This gentle movement can help increase your flexibility and strength without overwhelming your joints if done thoughtfully. The joy of watching your efforts flourish can bring a sense of peace and satisfaction, essential for emotional well-being.

To maximize the joy of gardening while minimizing strain on your body, consider a few important techniques. Start by selecting raised beds or container gardens. This can significantly reduce the need to bend over or kneel, making it easier on your back and knees. Choose pots or elevated surfaces at a comfortable height. When planting or weeding, it's helpful to use stools or kneelers with handles to aid in getting up and down, reducing the stress on your joints.

Always listen to your body and take breaks when needed. Gardening doesn't always need to be a marathon session; short, frequent periods of work may be less taxing and more enjoyable. Engaging in gentle stretches before and after gardening can help warm up your joints and prevent stiffness. Additionally, consider tools designed for those with arthritis, like ergonomically shaped hand tools or long-handled implements that provide extra leverage. These tools can reduce the strain on your hands and wrists, enabling you to garden longer and more comfortably. Remember, gardening should be a joy, not a chore, so make adjustments and create a space that feels good for you.

For anyone experiencing arthritis, it's important to keep your hydration levels up, especially when spending time outside. Keeping a water bottle nearby while you garden not only encourages you to stay hydrated but also gives you frequent moments to pause and enjoy the beauty around you. Small adjustments can lead to a greatly enriching gardening experience.

Creating a Relaxing Outdoor Space

Designing an outdoor space that encourages relaxation and enjoyment starts with understanding your personal preferences and needs. Take a moment to envision what relaxation means to you. Whether it's curling up with a good book, enjoying a leisurely cup of coffee, or simply soaking in the sun, your outdoor space should reflect that vision. Consider the layout and flow of the area. A cozy nook surrounded by lush greenery can provide a perfect retreat. Incorporate comfortable seating made from natural materials, like wood or bamboo, that invites you to unwind. Add soft cushions and throws for extra comfort and a personal touch. Think about the colors around you; soft, earthy tones inspire calmness, while vibrant flowers can uplift and invigorate. Use the space you have, whether it's a large yard or a small balcony, to create a sanctuary where you can escape the chaos of everyday life. Lighting plays a pivotal role as well—string lights or lanterns can transform your outdoor area into a magical haven during the evening hours.

Using elements of nature can significantly improve both mental and physical well-being. The sound of rustling leaves, chirping birds, and the gentle flow of water can create a soothing backdrop, reducing stress and promoting relaxation. Consider incorporating plants that resonate with you; aromatic herbs like lavender or mint not only smell wonderful but can also enhance your mood. If possible, add a water feature, such as a small fountain or birdbath, to engage your senses. The sight and sound of water can create a serene atmosphere, encouraging mindfulness and presence. Embrace the palette of nature—various greens, blues, and earthy tones can create harmony and balance in your space. Grounding yourself by walking barefoot on grass or soil connects you to the earth, allowing stress to dissipate. A mindful moment spent in nature, even in your own backyard, can become a powerful tool for your overall well-being. Taking time to breathe deeply and absorb your surroundings will invariably encourage a relaxed state of mind.

Creating a relaxing outdoor space is not just about aesthetics; it's a commitment to self-care and nurturing your spirit. Embrace the process of making your outdoor area a true reflection of what you need to feel at ease. A small daily practice, such as stepping outside for just a few minutes, can make a substantial difference in your day. This little act of stepping into nature can ground you, replenish your energy, and reframe your mindset, paving the way for a healthier, more balanced life.

Accessible Paths and Walkways

Creating safe and accessible pathways in outdoor spaces requires a thoughtful approach, one that considers the diverse needs of everyone who might use them. When I first began exploring the world through various landscapes, I noticed the barriers that could often arise—uneven surfaces, steep inclines, and narrow paths. These obstacles affect not just those with disabilities but anyone looking to enjoy these spaces, whether they are parents with strollers, older adults, or even those recovering from an injury. To truly foster inclusion, we must prioritize the design of our pathways. Utilizing materials that provide better traction and ensuring that surfaces are smooth can help everyone navigate these areas confidently. Moreover, attention to signage and lighting ensures that individuals can travel safely, day or night, feeling empowered rather than restricted by their environment. It's important to remember that every step we take toward creating accessible spaces brings us closer to a community where everyone can thrive.

Maintaining pathways is just as crucial as their initial creation. Regular maintenance and inspections can substantially reduce hazards that may develop over time. I've walked through areas where tree roots, erosion, or even water damage create dangerous conditions. Small cracks can quickly turn into larger issues, and if left unattended, they may discourage individuals from using these paths altogether. By incorporating routine checks and prompt repairs, we can ensure that pathways remain safe and welcoming. Additionally, community involvement can play a significant role. Encouraging locals to report issues or become involved in maintenance can foster a sense of ownership and responsibility toward these shared spaces. When individuals feel that these paths belong to them, it inspires a culture of care and respect that benefits all who use them.

There's a powerful connection between people and the environments we inhabit. Each accessible path we create and maintain not only improves physical access but also cultivates a sense of belonging. Whether it's through a stroll, a run, or a simple walk with loved ones, these pathways become avenues for connection. For those passionate about improving their communities, seeking partnerships with local organizations can be key. Many groups seek volunteers for clean-up days or improvement projects, creating opportunities to contribute to something greater. By harnessing these collaborative efforts, we can build a network of accessible paths that serve as lifelines for everyone. Remember, every action, no matter how small, contributes to a larger impact, making our spaces more navigable and enjoyable for all.

Outdoor Furniture Choices

Choosing outdoor furniture is not just a matter of style; it's about creating a space that invites comfort and enjoyment. When I first started looking for the perfect pieces for my patio, I quickly realized how essential it was to select furniture that felt good to use. You want to make sure that every chair, table, and lounger not only complements your outdoor décor but also offers a cozy spot to relax. It's about finding that sweet spot where aesthetics meet comfort. Look for pieces that fit your body well, allowing you and your loved ones to sink in and unwind after a long day. Try to envision yourself using the furniture – will you enjoy sitting in that chair for hours, or does it feel stiff and uninviting? Thoroughly testing out options is key; take those cushions for a test sit before making your purchase.

Prioritizing furniture that enhances outdoor enjoyment opens up a world of possibilities and encourages a lifestyle filled with more sunshine and fresh air. Imagine hosting friends for a barbecue, or spending quiet evenings with a partner under the stars, all while enveloped in the comfort of well-chosen pieces. Choose furniture that draws you outside and makes you want to linger in your backyard or garden. Surround yourself with colors and materials that resonate with nature, and invest in items that inspire connection – both with yourself and with others. The right outdoor furniture invites easy conversations, laughter, and moments of tranquility. It elevates your space and, in turn, enriches your life. Remember, investing in quality pieces is not merely about the purchase; it's about creating lasting memories in the space you've cultivated.

As you consider what outdoor furniture to bring into your world, think about how each choice fits into the lifestyle you aspire to lead. Whether you envision lavish dinners under the canopy of trees or quiet mornings sipping coffee, your selections will shape those experiences. Aim for pieces that resonate with you on a personal level, ensuring they aren't just functional but also bring a smile to your face. Always keep in mind that outdoor living can be a source of joy, relaxation, and connection – and your furniture choices play a vital role in that journey. To enhance your outdoor experience, consider integrating textural elements like soft rugs or cushions that can elevate comfort and style, making your outdoor area feel as inviting as the interiors of your home.

Safety Measures for Outdoor Activities

Engaging in outdoor activities brings a rush of excitement and a chance to connect with nature, but it is crucial to consider safety measures to protect yourself and those around you. Whether you are hiking, rock climbing, or biking, each activity presents unique challenges and potential hazards. For instance, ensuring you wear appropriate gear tailored to your specific activity can make a significant difference. Sturdy shoes, helmets, and weather-appropriate clothing are fundamental. It's also essential to carry a basic first aid kit and have a plan for emergencies. Before setting out, familiarize yourself with the terrain and weather conditions, as these can affect your experience and safety. Always inform someone about your plans, including the route you will take and the time you expect to return. This measure is a small but impactful way to ensure someone knows where you are in case things go awry.

Understanding and acknowledging personal limits is vital for anyone engaging in outdoor activities. Each of us has our own set of strengths and weaknesses, and it's okay to recognize them. Pushing beyond those limits can lead to accidents and injuries. During my early experiences outdoors, I found that listening to my body was just as important as following my adventurous spirit. Take breaks when you need them, stay hydrated, and do not hesitate to turn back if you feel uncomfortable or exhausted. Safe practices also involve learning the skills necessary for your chosen activity. For example, if you're venturing into climbing, take the time to understand the basics of equipment and safety protocols. Awareness not only enhances your safety but also uplifts others around you, creating a more secure environment for everyone involved.

One key tip to enhance your outdoor experiences is to engage with fellow enthusiasts or join local groups that focus on your activity of choice. Sharing experiences with others can provide insights into safe practices, help you stay accountable, and create a network of support. Many seasoned adventurers are more than willing to share their knowledge and experiences. Surrounding yourself with those who prioritize safety can inspire you to adopt these practices in your own adventures. Remember that embracing the joys of outdoor activities does not mean neglecting safety; it means combining your passion with prudence for a fulfilling experience.

Chapter 11: Lighting Solutions

Types of Lighting for Visibility

Exploring various types of lighting reveals how essential it is for visibility at home. Natural light is often the most effective, filling a room with warmth and clarity, making even the smallest details pop. However, we can't always rely on the sun's schedule. This is where artificial lighting comes in. Incandescent bulbs cast a cozy glow, perfect for relaxation, while LEDs offer bright, energy-efficient illumination ideal for tasks. Fluorescent lights can be a bit harsh but work well in spaces that require consistent lighting, like kitchens or home offices. Understanding how each of these types interacts with color and space can truly transform how we perceive our homes. Imagine the difference between a dimly lit corner and a spot flooded with soft, white light—you can feel the energy change, and so does the atmosphere around you.

Proper lighting plays a pivotal role in enhancing safety and comfort within our homes. It helps prevent accidents by illuminating stairways and hallways, ensuring we navigate spaces with ease. Well-lit environments reduce the risk of trips and falls, particularly for those who might feel uncertain in darker areas. Additionally, good lighting helps create a sense of security; knowing that each shadow is defined and that every corner is visible can keep anxieties at bay. Beyond safety, lighting affects our mood. A warm light can make a space feel inviting and cozy, perfect for unwinding after a long day, while bright, cool light can invigorate us, providing the energy needed for productivity. It's astounding how a simple switch can alter the ambiance of a room, contributing to our overall well-being.

When selecting lighting for your home, consider layering different types to create a versatile environment. Combining ambient, task, and accent lighting offers flexibility, allowing you to adjust the brightness based on your needs and activities. For instance, using dimmers can give you control over how alive or calm a room feels at different times of the day. Think about having a soft glow for evenings and brighter options for mornings when you need that burst of alertness. Experimenting with your lighting can lead to delightful discoveries about how your space can make you feel. A thoughtful approach to lighting can elevate not just visibility but also comfort within your sanctuary, making it a place where you feel truly at ease.

Adjustable and Motion Sensor Lights

Adjustable and motion sensor lighting options are becoming increasingly popular for many reasons, particularly for their convenience. In my own experience, I've found that installing these lights transforms how I interact with my home. Imagine walking into a room and having the lights automatically turn on as you step through the door, illuminating your path without a single touch. The convenience of not fumbling for a switch while carrying groceries or dealing with clutter can alleviate so much stress. These lights adapt not only to your movements but also to your needs, whether it's setting a gentle glow for a late-night snack or brightening a space when you have guests. It's about creating an environment that supports your lifestyle and enhances the comfort of your surroundings.

The benefits of energy efficiency and ease of use are undeniable. With traditional lighting, I often found myself leaving lights on in rooms I no longer occupied, unaware of how much energy was being wasted. Motion sensor lights address this issue effortlessly; they turn off automatically after no movement is detected for a set period. This feature not only conserves energy but also saves money on utility bills—a win-win scenario! Additionally, adjustable lighting allows you to customize the intensity of light based on the time of day or activity at hand. Whether you're reading, entertaining, or simply relaxing, having the right lighting can significantly enhance the atmosphere and your overall experience. The design of these lights can cater to anyone's style while improving energy efficiency, proving that practical solutions can also be aesthetically pleasing.

Ultimately, embracing adjustable and motion sensor lights is about more than just convenience. It reflects a lifestyle choice aimed at reducing our environmental footprint while improving daily functionality. When you're engaged in life and always on the go, let your home respond to your needs effortlessly—this transition not only simplifies your space but also contributes positively to the planet. A practical tip for anyone considering this upgrade is to evaluate the specific areas in your home where motion sensors would be most beneficial, such as hallways, bathrooms, or outside entrances. This targeted approach ensures you maximize the benefits of these lighting solutions while creating a safer, more functional living space.

Eliminating Shadows and Glare

Arranging lighting to minimize shadows and control glare in your home starts with understanding the different sources of light and how they interact within your space. Natural light can create dynamic experiences, but it can also lead to unwanted glare, especially when it hits reflective surfaces. Introducing layered lighting, which combines ambient, task, and accent lights, can help to create a balance. Use lamps with shades that diffuse the light to soften harsh brightness and reduce the starkness that causes shadows. Positioning light sources thoughtfully can also make a significant difference. For example, placing a lamp to the side and slightly behind where you'll be reading can improve visibility without creating shadows that line your face. When working under overhead lights, consider using dimmers to adjust brightness levels, allowing you to tailor the environment to your activities and needs.

A well-lit environment enhances focus and safety, crucial for maintaining motivation and productivity in your day-to-day life. Think about creating different zones in your home, where each area is illuminated according to its purpose. For instance, a bright workspace encourages creativity—using daylight bulbs can be particularly effective. In contrast, softer lighting in relaxation areas promotes calmness and comfort. Additionally, enhancing safety means considering lighting pathways and dark corners, especially in homes with stairs or multiple levels. Motion sensor lights can automatically illuminate these areas when movement is detected, creating a welcoming and secure atmosphere day or night. Having intentional lighting not only supports your activities but also aids in your overall well-being, leading to a more vibrant experience in your space.

Before making significant changes, start small. Experiment with different types of light bulbs, adjusting their positions and intensities until you find what feels best for you. A simple tryout by repositioning your current lamps can lead to noticeable improvements. You might find that a cozy corner becomes your favorite reading nook with just a little tweak. Continuous adjustments will help you develop an intuitive understanding of how light influences your mood and productivity. Remember, the goal is to create an environment where every space feels inviting, energizing, and safe.

Smart Home Lighting Technologies

Smart lighting technologies are transforming the way we interact with our living spaces, providing a unique blend of convenience and adaptability that caters to our modern lifestyles. Imagine coming home after a long day, and as you step through the door, the lights automatically brighten to your favorite warm hue. This isn't just a luxury; it's part of a wave of advancements designed to enhance comfort and efficiency in our homes. With smart bulbs and systems connected via apps on our smartphones, controlling the ambiance becomes as easy as a swipe or a voice command. Not only do these technologies reduce the need to fumble around for switches, but they can also learn our habits over time, adjusting automatically to our preferences. The result is a home that feels inherently more inviting and responsive to our needs, creating a haven of ease in a hectic world.

For individuals with mobility challenges, smart lighting offers an essential advantage that can significantly improve daily life. Accessing traditional switches can be cumbersome, if not impossible, but with the advent of smart controls, the barriers are greatly diminished. Voice-activated systems allow you to command your lights without lifting a finger. Whether it's through smart assistants like Amazon Alexa or Google Home, the control over your environment is in your voice. Imagine being able to adjust your lighting from the comfort of your chair or bed, making it a seamless part of your day rather than a challenge. This ease of control demystifies the home environment and allows users to feel empowered, fostering independence and comfort in spaces where they can truly be themselves.

The integration of these technologies not only enhances convenience but also promotes a more inclusive ethos within our homes. By understanding how these tools can create positive changes, we open ourselves to a world of possibilities that can meet everyone's unique needs. As we continue to embrace innovation in our living spaces, let's remember to explore the features that smart lighting offers, such as scheduling, energy efficiency, and mood settings. Experimenting with different combinations can lead to delightful discoveries that enhance well-being and create a warm, welcoming atmosphere. A simple tip to get started is to choose one room in your home to set up smart lighting. This not only eases you into the technology but also sets the stage for a transformation that can elevate your daily experience.

Creating Ambiance and Comfort

Using lighting techniques to create a warm and inviting ambience in your home reveals a transformative power that can completely change how a space feels. Just imagine walking into a room where your eyes are greeted by soft, warm hues rather than harsh, glaring lights. Incorporating different layers of lighting, like ambient, task, and accent, can turn your living space into a sanctuary. Start with the kind of light bulbs you choose; warm white bulbs, typically around 2700K, give off a cozy glow that feels inviting. Consider placing them in lamps that disperse light gently, rather than the exposed bulbs that can create an uncomfortable glare.

Strategically placing lights can also play with the spatial perception of a room. Soft lighting in corners, for example, can draw the eye and make a room feel wider and more expansive. Arrange your furniture to allow light to filter through, perhaps using mirrors to bounce warmth back into the room. It's all about crafting a space that feels both personal and comfortable, a space where you truly want to linger.

The psychological effects of lighting on mood and comfort cannot be underestimated. Light impacts our emotions more than we might realize. Bright, harsh lights can evoke feelings of anxiety or stress, whereas soft, muted lighting can promote feelings of calm and relaxation. When you set the right atmosphere, it encourages us to unwind and feel at home. This intrinsic connection between light and mood is essential, especially in areas where you seek rest, like your bedroom or living room. Be mindful of how you curate your space. A well-lit area can uplift spirits, foster conversations, and create bonds. To achieve this, consider dimmer switches or smart home devices that allow you to adjust lighting throughout the day. This flexibility enables you to align with your natural rhythms, creating a comforting retreat where you can truly nourish your soul.

A practical tip to enhance the ambiance in your home is to incorporate multiple light sources at different heights. This approach creates a layered effect, leading to a fuller, more inviting environment. The next time you rearrange or update a space, think about the various ways light dances around. Your home can be more than just a place to rest; it can be a haven of comfort and warmth.

Chapter 12: Temperature Control

Importance of Temperature Regulation

Temperature has a profound impact on arthritis symptoms and our overall comfort. On chilly days, I often feel the stiffness creeping into my joints, each step reminding me of the struggles I face. Cold can tighten our muscles and exacerbate the pain we experience. Likewise, heat can be equally troublesome. While warm temperatures may feel soothing, they can lead to swelling and discomfort if the environment is too humid or warm. Everyone's sensitivity to temperature can vary, and understanding our own bodies is crucial. Learning how my joints respond to different climates has empowered me to take control of my comfort levels.

Creating a comfortable home environment becomes essential when navigating these physical challenges. It's not just about adjusting the thermostat; it's about crafting a sanctuary where comfort reigns, and pain takes a back seat. Consider investing in blankets that retain warmth during cold months, or air conditioning systems that keep the heat at bay. Beyond temperature control, the little things—like a comfortable chair to ease joint pain or keeping the living space organized—influence how we feel in our surroundings. Enhancing our home environment can help create a supportive atmosphere that encourages relaxation and well-being.

Make it a habit to monitor your environment and adjust settings according to your needs. For instance, wearing layers can help you manage temperature fluctuations throughout the day, and adding a humidifier can balance air moisture during dry months. This thoughtful attention to temperature can significantly enhance your quality of life. Each moment spent in a comfortable setting is a moment where we can focus on things that truly matter instead of being sidelined by discomfort.

Heating Solutions for Comfort

As the temperature drops, finding ways to keep your home cozy and comfortable becomes essential. Various heating solutions exist to cater to different needs and preferences. Central heating systems are popular for whole-home warmth, circulating heated air through ductwork. For those looking for localized warmth, space heaters are great options. These come in electric and gas varieties and can easily be moved from room to room. Radiant floor heating is another luxurious choice, allowing warmth to rise from the floor, making chilly mornings feel significantly more pleasant. Don't overlook fireplaces and wood stoves, which provide not only heat but also a beautiful ambiance that instantly creates a welcoming environment.

When selecting the best heating option, several factors should guide your choice. First, consider the size and layout of your home. A larger space may require more robust solutions, while smaller areas could benefit from compact heaters. Energy efficiency is significant too; opting for systems with high-efficiency ratings can save you money on utility bills and reduce your carbon footprint. Think about your lifestyle as well—if you're often away from home, programmable thermostats can optimize your heating schedule. Finally, don't forget to factor in maintenance and installation costs, as these will influence your long-term satisfaction with the heating solution you choose.

As you navigate the options available, remember that the ultimate goal is to create a sanctuary that shields you from the cold while promoting relaxation and comfort. It can be helpful to consult with a heating expert who understands your specific situation and can guide you through the myriad of choices. Taking the time to select the right heating system can transform your home into a true haven during the colder months, ensuring that every corner feels inviting.

Cooling Options During Hot Weather

Finding ways to cool down during sweltering summer days can feel like a daunting task, especially when temperatures rise and sweat seems to cling to every surface. One of the simplest yet effective solutions is to embrace the power of airflow. Opening windows and allowing a gentle breeze to enter, particularly in the early morning or late evening hours, can help create a natural current that reduces indoor temperatures. Ceiling fans and portable fans can further enhance this effect. Not only do they add movement to the air, but they also help evaporate sweat from our skin, making us feel cooler without significantly lowering the room temperature.

In addition to enhancing airflow, it's essential to consider how our homes manage humidity levels during the heat. High humidity can make a warm day feel stifling, amplifying discomfort. One effective strategy is to keep blinds or curtains closed during peak sunlight hours. This simple act can shield your living space from the harsh rays of the sun and significantly reduce indoor temperatures. Using heat-reflective or blackout drapes can further enhance this benefit. Another crucial element is to maintain proper ventilation and air circulation within the house. Installing exhaust fans in areas like the kitchen and bathroom can help remove excess humidity, while also preventing it from building up in other areas of the home. Dehumidifiers can also work wonders, making the air feel cooler and more comfortable.

By approaching the heat with a blend of these strategies, we can create a welcoming oasis in our homes, shielding ourselves from the summer blaze. Moreover, embracing the use of plants indoors not only beautifies the space but also helps regulate humidity levels naturally. Plants release moisture into the air through a process called transpiration, and certain varieties, like peace lilies and spider plants, are particularly skilled at improving air quality. So as you seek refuge from the heat, remember that every small action—whether it's adjusting a fan or nurturing a houseplant—can bring relief and transform your living space into a cool, refreshing retreat.

Humidity and its Effects on Arthritis

Humidity levels can significantly influence arthritis symptoms and comfort. Many people with arthritis often find that their joints feel particularly stiff and painful when humidity is high. This might seem surprising, but the changes in atmospheric pressure that accompany higher humidity can exacerbate inflammation in the joints. When the air is heavy with moisture, it seems to affect everyone differently, but for those of us managing arthritis, it can feel like a weight pressing down on our bones. You might notice that rainy days bring more discomfort, and as the humidity climbs, your joints may ache more than usual. These changes can lead to a frustrating cycle where the weather dictates how well we can move and enjoy our lives, making mundane tasks feel like monumental challenges.

It's important, therefore, to monitor and manage the humidity levels in your environment for improved well-being. Using a hygrometer can help track indoor humidity, allowing you to take measures to maintain a comfortable level. If it's too humid, air conditioning or dehumidifiers can reduce moisture in the air, creating a more arthritis-friendly atmosphere. On the other hand, if the air is too dry, especially during winter months, using a humidifier can keep your joints moist and ease discomfort. Taking such proactive steps not only enhances comfort but can also empower you to regain some control over your arthritis. Remember, adjusting your environment can lead to greater mobility and an improved quality of life.

As you manage the humidity levels around you, don't forget the small but impactful choices that contribute to your overall health. Staying well-hydrated is crucial;

it helps maintain the lubrication in your joints independent of the outside conditions. Consider incorporating gentle exercises or stretches into your routine, which can also help maintain your joint function despite the weather. Knowledge and adjustment of your environment can create a more comfortable space, allowing you to focus on the activities you enjoy and enhancing your journey with arthritis.

Smart Thermostats for Ease of Use

Smart thermostats represent a significant leap forward in how we manage our home environments. They bring efficient temperature control right to our fingertips. Imagine coming home after a long day and walking into a space that feels just right, not too hot and not too cold. With smart thermostats, this is not just a luxury; it's an everyday possibility. Equipped with advanced sensors and intelligent algorithms, these devices learn your habits over time. They adjust temperatures based on your routines, ensuring that your home is always comfortable without wasting energy. It's remarkable how such a small device can make a big difference in our daily lives, making every return home a pleasant experience.

The convenience of remote control is another compelling reason to embrace smart thermostats. Through a user-friendly app on your smartphone or tablet, you can make adjustments from anywhere. Have you ever left home on a scorching summer day only to realize you forgot to turn down the air conditioning? With a smart thermostat, you can quickly switch it on, no matter where you are. This feature not only adds comfort but also enhances energy efficiency. You can monitor and adjust energy use in real time, making informed choices that lower your utility bills. It's about being in control and having peace of mind, knowing that your home environment is taken care of, even when you're miles away.

As you consider adopting this technology, think about the possibilities it brings to your life. Not only does it enhance your living experience, but it also contributes to a more sustainable lifestyle. Smart thermostats enable you to reduce your carbon footprint while enjoying ultimate comfort. They are designed to adapt to your needs, making it easier for you to create an environment that feels just right. Don't hesitate to explore the features of smart thermostats and make the switch; you'll likely find this small change leads to significant benefits in your daily routine. Start by looking for a device that fits your needs and consider how it can simplify your life.

Chapter 13: Organizational Strategies

Decluttering Your Home

Decluttering can be a transformative experience, especially for those living with arthritis. When I started my decluttering journey, I quickly realized that the impact went beyond just having more space. Physically, a clean and organized home reduces the chance of stumbling over clutter, minimizing the risk of falls and injuries that can be detrimental for those with joint pain. Each removed item felt like I was shedding a weight that had been lingering on both my body and mind. It was liberating.

Mentally, the act of decluttering creates a sense of control and accomplishment. Arthritis can often make us feel helpless, so reclaiming our living space can reignite a sense of empowerment. The process itself is engaging; as we make choices about what to keep and what to let go, we foster a stronger connection to our environment. This is crucial, as emotional well-being can significantly influence our physical health. The increased clarity and focus that comes from organizing your space can lead to reduced stress levels, allowing for better management of arthritis symptoms.

Cultivating an organized living space starts with small, manageable steps. When I decided to take on this challenge, I prioritized one room at a time. Focusing on a single area not only made the process feel less overwhelming but also allowed me to witness the immediate benefits of my efforts. Start by designating a specific time each week to work on decluttering. Even just 15 to 20 minutes can lead to significant progress over time.

As you sort through items, ask yourself questions that center around their necessity and functionality. Consider whether an item adds value to your life or simply creates noise in your space. Involving your family members in the process can also create a sense of teamwork, making it a shared experience rather than a chore. Labeling boxes or bins helps create a sense of order when organizing what to keep, donate, or discard, especially in spaces like the kitchen or living room where clutter tends to build up quickly. It's eye-opening to see how much we can let go of when we take the time to evaluate our possessions with intention.

Finally, create a designated space for things that are frequently used. This makes accessing everyday items easier and reduces the physical strain that comes with searching through clutter. Consider keeping a small basket for essential items that need to be stowed away after use. Even these small changes can enhance your living space and well-being profoundly, making it feel both functional and serene.

Finding time for decluttering amidst the challenges of arthritis can be a journey, but it's worth it. I encourage you to start with just one small area. You might be surprised by how much lighter and more energized you feel afterward.

Creating Systematic Storage Solutions

Developing organizational systems that enhance accessibility and usability can transform the way we navigate our spaces. When I embarked on creating my own storage solutions, I realized that the key was not just to have a place for everything, but to have everything in a place that made sense. Every time I opened a drawer or a cabinet, I wanted to feel a sense of relief instead of frustration. So, I started categorizing items by their frequency of use. The things I needed daily went in easy-to-reach spots, while seasonal or rarely used items were placed higher up or further back. This approach not only simplified my daily routines but also made the space feel more inviting. Finding what I needed became a breeze, bringing a wonderful sense of calm to my home.

Systematic storage solutions contribute significantly to reducing the need for excessive reaching or bending, which is crucial for our physical well-being, especially as we grow older. I've experienced firsthand how a well-thought-out system can ease stress on the body. For instance, I made a conscious effort to keep frequently used kitchen items at waist level. No more awkward twisting or stretching to grab a spice jar tucked out of reach. By keeping things at an accessible height, I found that my back and joints felt much better after a long day. Additionally, I began implementing pull-out shelves in my cabinets. This simple change allowed me to access items in the back without contorting myself and saved me from potential strains or injuries.

Implementing these systematic storage solutions was more than just making my home functional; it was about fostering an environment that promotes ease and comfort. It's incredible how little changes in how we store our belongings can significantly improve our daily life experience. A practical tip is to utilize clear bins or labels so that you can easily see where everything belongs. Not only does this enhance organization, but it also allows you to save time and energy when looking for items. Remember, a well-structured space doesn't just clean up clutter; it clears the mind.

Labeling and Accessibility

Labeling plays a crucial role in our daily lives, serving as a meaningful bridge between us and the items we need. From a simple jar of jam in the pantry to complex medical supplies in a hospital, the purpose of a label is clear: to provide immediate recognition and facilitate access. Imagine standing in front of a cluttered shelf, seeking your favorite spices. Clear labels cut through the chaos, granting you swift access to what you desire. When I reorganized my kitchen and added labels, I found myself spending less time searching and more time enjoying the cooking process. Every can, box, and bottle had a clear identity, leading to a more efficient and harmonious space. This simple act of labeling transformed my routine, allowing me to focus on what truly matters—preparing nourishing meals for my loved ones.

Clear labels do more than enhance our ability to find items; they significantly ease our mental load. I recall a time when I was feeling overwhelmed trying to locate essential documents in a stack of papers. My stress compounded with each fruitless attempt to search through disorganized chaos, heightening my sense of frustration. However, implementing a labeling system to categorize those documents changed everything. No longer did I waste precious energy combing through piles of uncertainty. Each labeled folder displayed its contents prominently, guiding me straight to what I needed. This newfound ease not only saved me time but also reduced the physical and emotional strain of searching. Whether in our homes, workplaces, or even within our minds, clear labels create a pathway for clarity, allowing us to navigate effortlessly and with confidence.

Consider the environments you frequent, and the items you often need. Take a moment to reflect on how a simple label could enhance your ability to locate what you require without the burden of unnecessary effort. Bringing organization through labeling can transform your space and, indeed, your day-to-day life.

Incorporating Vertical Space

Embracing vertical space has been a game-changer in my quest for a more organized life. It became clear to me that the walls of my home were an untapped resource just waiting to be utilized. I started by assessing each room, identifying where I could add shelves or hooks. For instance, in my kitchen, I mounted shelves above the counter to store jars of spices and cooking utensils, freeing up precious counter space. I found that using vertical storage not only reduced the clutter that usually occupied my countertops but also made everything easily accessible. Simple items like floating shelves or over-the-door racks can do wonders, allowing you to elevate your belongings and creating a more breathable atmosphere around you.   Making the most of vertical space doesn't stop at traditional shelving. I looked into using stackable storage bins that I could place at higher levels in closets and garages. These bins helped keep seasonal items or seldom-used tools out of the way, yet easily reachable when necessary. With a little creativity, I transformed empty wall space into functional areas for displaying art, plants, or books. It turned my living space into a reflection of my personality while channeling my clutter into organized sections.

Once I realized the potential of vertical space, the next step was to manage items in ways that significantly improved functionality and accessibility. A pivotal moment for me was rethinking the purpose of the items I owned. Instead of seeing a collection of things to be stored, I began viewing them as tools to create a harmonious living environment. For instance, I grouped similar items together and placed them on designated shelves, like combining all my cooking books and materials onto one high shelf in the kitchen. This not only kept things neat but made it so much easier to find what I needed.   I also introduced multifunctional furniture into my living spaces. A bench with storage underneath became a great addition to my entryway, where I could not only sit while putting on shoes but also store shopping bags and seasonal gear simultaneously. I became attuned to the equations of space and function, finding ways to incorporate items that serve multiple purposes.   It's essential to remember that maintaining an organized space takes continual effort and reflection. Regularly revisiting and adjusting these systems has been crucial in minimizing clutter and improving overall functionality. As a practical tip, consider setting aside a few moments each week to reassess how you're using your vertical space. It can be as simple as shifting a few decorative pieces around or swapping out items based on seasonality. This ongoing adjustment keeps your space dynamic and aligned with your current lifestyle. Finding balance and beauty in organization can be a rewarding journey that not only transforms your space but also revitalizes your spirit.

Daily Maintenance Routines

Establishing daily routines is crucial to maintaining an organized and accessible home. It's easy to let messes accumulate, especially with the busyness of everyday life. I remember when I first realized the impact of small, consistent actions. After a long day, coming home to a cluttered space left me feeling stressed and overwhelmed. By simply dedicating a few minutes each day to tidying up, I noticed a significant change. Everything from the kitchen counters to the living room began to feel more inviting. Routines help create a sense of order, allowing us to navigate our homes with ease. When everything has its place, we can find what we need quickly, improving our overall mood and productivity. It's amazing how a little effort each day can build a sanctuary that feels calm and restful instead of chaotic and draining.

Involving family members in daily maintenance can amplify the positive effects of these routines. I found that when I included my family in the process, it not only lightened my load but also fostered a sense of teamwork and responsibility. Encouraging everyone to contribute, whether it's picking up their own items or participating in shared chores, cultivates a spirit of collaboration. It creates an environment where everyone feels invested in our home. Plus, tackling tasks together often leads to laughter and bonding time, making chores feel less laborious. By setting expectations and making it a family affair, we transform responsibilities into moments of connection, reinforcing the idea that our home is a shared space that thrives on collective effort.

To make these daily routines stick, you might want to assign specific roles or create a simple chore chart. This gives everyone clarity and accountability while also breaking down larger tasks into manageable bits. Don't hesitate to celebrate the little victories, too. Whether it's a clean kitchen sink or an uncluttered living room, acknowledging these successes can boost motivation and reinforce the habit. Remember, building a routine is a journey that takes time and patience, but the peace of mind that comes from a well-maintained home is worth every effort.

Chapter 14: Safety Precautions

Identifying Home Hazards

Identifying potential hazards within your home environment begins with a careful examination of the spaces where you live and interact daily. It's important to look beyond just the visible risks; many hazards may be lurking beneath the surface or in everyday items. For example, check for frayed electrical cords, which pose a fire risk, or assess the stability of shelves and furniture that could topple over. Paying attention to slips and falls is crucial. Look for uneven flooring, loose rugs, or cluttered walkways that might cause accidents. Remember to consider less obvious dangers as well, like carbon monoxide leaks from gas appliances or mold creeping in damp areas. These hidden threats can often go unnoticed but can have serious implications for the health and safety of your loved ones. By conducting a thorough walkthrough of your home and creating a systematic approach to hazard identification, you set the stage for a safer living environment.

Taking the time to address any identified hazards is not just a matter of preference; it's an essential part of caring for those who reside in your home. Each potential risk you eliminate contributes not only to physical safety but also to peace of mind. It can be easy to become overwhelmed when faced with a list of improvements, yet remember that every small step counts. Begin with the most pressing issues and work your way to others, and draw on the support of family or friends if necessary. Engaging in this process together can strengthen relationships as you share the common goal of safety. Holding yourself accountable and ensuring that your home is a sanctuary of safety isn't just a responsibility; it's a profound way to express love and care. Your attentive efforts to mitigate hazards show those around you that their well-being is your top priority.

When you take hazard identification seriously, you are not only protecting your physical surroundings but also nurturing the emotional and mental health of everyone in your home. A safe environment promotes relaxation and happiness, free from the anxiety of what lurks in the shadows. As you commit to the journey of making your home safer, don't forget the importance of regular check-ins. Home safety is not a one-time task; it's an ongoing process that requires you to stay vigilant and proactive. Make it a routine to assess your space, update safety measures, and discuss concerns with your household regularly. This can be as simple as setting aside a few minutes each month to walk through and check key areas. Safety in the home is a journey, and every step you take makes a tangible difference.

Emergency Preparedness Plans

Having an emergency plan is crucial for anyone, but for those of us living with arthritis, it takes on a special urgency. Arthritis can be unpredictable. Flare-ups, pain, and fatigue can strike at any moment, which makes it challenging to respond effectively in emergencies. This unpredictability is why we cannot afford to be caught unprepared. An emergency plan helps ensure that our unique needs are met, allowing us to navigate crises with a little less stress.

When you have a plan, you know what to do, and that knowledge can ease anxiety. I remember a time when my arthritis flared up unexpectedly during a severe weather alert. I had no idea what to do, and it left me feeling vulnerable. If I had had a solid plan in place, I could have focused on my condition rather than worrying about potential dangers. Having an emergency plan helps keep our minds clear and focused, giving us the confidence to handle whatever might come our way.

Creating an accessible emergency response plan requires thoughtful consideration about our specific needs. Start by identifying what triggers your arthritis symptoms and how these might limit your ability to react in an emergency. For instance, if mobility is an issue, ensure you have a clear path to an exit, free of barriers. Involve family members or caregivers in this process, as they can provide invaluable support and insights into your situation.

Make sure your emergency contacts are easy to reach. Have a list of those you can call in case you need assistance, and ensure these contacts are aware of your needs. Practice scenarios where you might need to rely on them, so they know how best to help you. Writing down essential information like medication schedules, allergies, and medical history can also be a lifesaver in emergencies. Keep this information in a secure yet easily accessible place, both at home and on your phone.

Finally, it's beneficial to rehearse your emergency plan. Practice might sound tedious, but it pays off when every second counts. You'll feel more prepared, and when the moment comes, your response will feel seamless rather than reactive. This proactive approach reduces anxiety and empowers you to face emergencies with strength. Remember, the goal is to make the plan work for you, and don't hesitate to update it as your needs change.

One practical tip that can make a huge difference is to create a 'go bag'—a bag filled with essentials you might need during an emergency, such as medications, water, and snacks suitable for your diet. Including a copy of your emergency plan can transform your preparation from a daunting task into an action you can take with ease.

First Aid and Arthritis Management

Understanding how to approach first-aid for arthritis-related issues is crucial for anyone dealing with this condition. When arthritis flares up, the pain can be severe and overwhelming. It's important to remember that while you may feel isolated in these moments, there are effective techniques that can help alleviate your discomfort. Applying a cold pack can significantly reduce swelling and numb the pain. Ensure to wrap the pack in a cloth to avoid ice burns. Alternatively, if your joints feel stiff, a warm compress can help increase circulation and relieve tension. It's also beneficial to position your joints in a comfortable way to minimize strain. Simple movements like stretching or gentle bending can help ease stiffness, but always listen to your body—never push beyond what feels okay. If you experience a sudden increase in pain or if your joint is hot or swollen, it may be necessary to seek professional medical help.

Preparedness is key when managing arthritis flare-ups. Having a plan establishes a sense of control during those unpredictable moments. Having essential items readily available, such as pain relief medication, heat and cold packs, and even supportive braces, can ease the immediate impact of a flare-up. It's also helpful to maintain an open line of communication with your healthcare provider or therapist to discuss any modifications to your treatment plan. Consider keeping a journal to track your flare-ups, noting what activities preceded them and how you managed the pain. This can be motivating, as you will begin to recognize patterns in your symptoms and responses. Remember that it's okay to ask for assistance; whether it's from family, friends, or healthcare providers, surrounding yourself with support can turn a challenging situation into a manageable one.

Ultimately, when it comes to arthritis care, empowerment and compassion for oneself are essential. Understanding your body and what it needs during a flare-up can make all the difference. Consider exploring relaxation techniques. Mindfulness, deep breathing, or guided imagery can help ease anxiety and stress, which often exacerbate pain. Approach each flare-up with patience and self-kindness. As you continue through this journey, keep in mind that even small actions can lead to improved outcomes. Always stay prepared, utilize the resources at your fingertips, and above all, be gentle with yourself as you navigate the ups and downs of living with arthritis.

Establishing Safe Zones

Establishing safe zones in your home is essential for creating a comfortable environment that supports both mobility and independence. When I first started thinking about my own space, I realized that having areas specifically designed for my needs made a world of difference. It's more than just rearranging furniture; it's about designing a physical space that empowers you. These zones should be free from obstacles, ensuring that you can move freely without risk. Start by assessing the areas you use most often, like the living room, kitchen, or bedroom. Identify any hazards and remove them. For instance, keeping pathways clear and using non-slip mats can help prevent falls.

Incorporating tools and furniture designed for ease of use is key. Consider investing in grab bars, raised toilet seats, or adjustable furniture. These modifications may seem small, but they significantly enhance your comfort and security. You can also use visual cues, such as painter's tape, to mark safe walking paths or indicate where to place furniture. Creating an environment that accommodates mobility needs allows you to access your space with confidence, facilitating participation in daily activities and interactions with loved ones. All of this contributes to a sense of control over your surroundings.

Having a personal safe space helps create a sanctuary where you feel secure both physically and mentally. I found that when I had a designated space just for me—where I could sit quietly, reflect, or simply breathe—my stress levels significantly decreased. Psychological benefits include enhanced feelings of safety and reduced anxiety. When you know you have a place to retreat to, it fosters a sense of autonomy, enabling you to handle challenges more effectively. The mere act of physically defining your space helps you regain control over your environment.

Moreover, these safe zones can encourage mindfulness and self-care, strengthening your emotional resilience. When I took time in my safe space for activities like reading or meditating, I noticed improvements in my overall well-being. The concept of personal space goes beyond just physical boundaries; it's about creating an oasis where you can recharge, reflect, and revitalize. A personal safe zone fosters not only peace of mind but also physical rejuvenation, reminding you of the importance of prioritizing your own needs amid life's hustle. Take those small steps today to carve out a safe space for yourself. Perhaps choose a corner of your room, adorn it with a cozy chair, and fill it with items that bring you joy. Your personal sanctuary awaits.

Assistive Devices for Safety

Assistive devices play a crucial role in enhancing safety within our homes. As someone who has navigated the challenges of living with a desire for greater independence, I've learned how vital these tools can be. They can transform spaces that once felt risky into environments where we can thrive. Simple modifications can make daily tasks more manageable, reducing anxiety and providing a sense of security. Whether it's a grab bar in the bathroom to prevent slips or a stair lift to navigate multi-level homes, these devices can help us maintain our dignity while ensuring safety. Embracing the right assistive devices can make a profound difference in our quality of life, allowing us to focus on what truly matters—enjoying our daily activities without the looming fear of accidents.

There are a range of aids designed to support our safety at home, each with its unique benefits. For instance, non-slip mats are excellent for bathrooms where water can create hazards. They provide stability and peace of mind, allowing us to step in and out with confidence. Similarly, motion sensor lights can illuminate dark hallways or staircases, eliminating the fear of falling while moving about at night. Kitchen aids, like reachers or easy-grip utensils, can help those with mobility limitations continue to prepare meals without straining. Remember, the goal is not only to reduce risks but also to empower ourselves to carry out our daily routines seamlessly. Even small changes, like ensuring that frequently used items are within easy reach, can significantly enhance our safety and independence.

One practical tip that can easily be implemented is to create a safety checklist for your home. Take a walk through your living space and identify areas that may require modifications. Consider factors like lighting, flooring, and the layout of furniture. Engage family members or caregivers in this process to gain valuable insights and support. By making these adjustments mindfully, you can cultivate a home that feels safer and more welcoming. Every step taken toward enhancing safety is not just an improvement in your environment but a profound commitment to your well-being.

Chapter 15: Technology Integration

Smart Home Devices and Control

Smart home devices are designed to simplify daily tasks, especially for those of us living with arthritis.

These devices can serve as helpful companions, making our lives easier and more manageable. Imagine waking up in the morning and having your coffee maker start brewing your favorite blend with just a simple command. Voice-controlled devices like smart speakers can help you set reminders or play your favorite music without any need for physical effort. Smart thermostats can adjust the temperature in your home, ensuring your comfort without the hassle of dealing with knobs or buttons that may be difficult to manage. Even smart lighting systems allow you to control brightness and set schedules from your phone or with voice commands, creating an inviting environment without putting strain on your joints.

Exploring technology that encourages independence is vital. Many smart devices come with user-friendly interfaces designed for ease of use, allowing men and women with arthritis to maintain a sense of control and autonomy in their daily lives. Whether it's a smart lock that lets you secure your home without the need for a key, or a smart appliance that can be programmed to meet your needs, these innovations show how technology can empower those dealing with mobility challenges. Adopting such technology not only simplifies everyday tasks but can also improve your overall well-being by fostering independence and reducing the frustration that often accompanies daily routines. Embracing this technological help can lead to greater confidence and a more fulfilling lifestyle.

Consider starting with just one device that piques your interest, whether it's a voice assistant or a smart plug. Take your time to explore what works best for you and see how it can fit seamlessly into your life. Little steps towards integrating smart technology can lead to significant improvements in your daily life, helping you reclaim your time and enjoy your independence once again.

Using Voice Assistants for Ease

Voice assistants have transformed the way we manage our daily tasks, easing the burden of our busy lives. Imagine stepping into your home after a long day, and with just your voice, you can adjust the lights to a warm glow, set your favorite playlist, and even ask for the weather forecast. This technology enables you to multitask effortlessly, allowing you to cook dinner while dictating a shopping list or setting reminders for important appointments. Every little convenience counts, especially when life moves at such a frenetic pace.

Using voice commands takes away the physical strain of managing devices. For example, instead of searching around for your phone or getting up to adjust the thermostat, you can simply speak your commands. This is particularly invaluable for those who might have mobility issues, creating a more inclusive and accessible environment within their homes. The engagement increases when technology meets empathy; these assistants are designed to simplify your life, making home management feel less intimidating and more enjoyable.

Accessibility is a significant benefit of voice technology that often goes unnoticed until it directly impacts our daily lives. For those who may struggle with traditional interfaces, voice assistants provide a simple, efficient alternative. This technology allows everyone, regardless of their physical capabilities, to interact with smart home features, manage appointments, and even seek information without relying on others. It empowers individuals to take back control over their environments, fostering a sense of independence that is often hard to achieve in today's fast-paced world.

Moreover, the convenience of having a personal assistant that is available 24/7 cannot be overstated. Whether you're settling into bed and remembering that you need to build a new playlist for a special occasion, or you're halfway through a workout and need to track your achievements, voice assistants keep your life seamlessly organized. They can learn your preferences, making future interactions even smoother. This sense of ease is not just beneficial, but it motivates individuals to embrace organization in all areas of their lives, leading to less stress and greater satisfaction.

To make the most of this technology, consider integrating voice assistants into your daily routine. Set specific reminders, manage your calendar with ease, or even utilize them for meal planning and recipe management. Embracing these tools isn't just about convenience; it's about enhancing your quality of life, allowing you to focus on what truly matters.

Health Monitoring Devices

Living with arthritis brings about unique challenges, and monitoring our health metrics has become imperative in managing this condition. Various devices are now available that can help track essential factors, such as joint inflammation, pain levels, physical activity, and even stress. For instance, smart wearables, like fitness trackers or smartwatches, can monitor our physical activity levels, reminding us to move when we've been stationary for too long. Some devices even feature customizable reminders to take medication, ensuring we don't forget the crucial steps needed for managing our symptoms. These gadgets can be an integral part of our daily routine, making it easier to remain aware of how our bodies are reacting to different activities and environments.

Furthermore, technology significantly aids in proactively managing symptoms. Many health monitoring devices sync with mobile applications, allowing us to visualize our performance over time. For example, recording pain levels daily in a simple app can reveal patterns that may prompt necessary changes in our routines or treatment plans. Some devices even include features that analyze sleep quality, which is vital for overall well-being and can be compromised by arthritis. By understanding how our bodies respond to various triggers, we can develop a more tailored approach to managing our health. In turn, this empowers us, fostering a sense of control over our lives rather than feeling at the mercy of our condition.

Take the time to explore and find the right tools that resonate with you. A simple step might be using a pain diary, whether physical or digital, to jot down how you feel each day. Tracking those details may help illustrate your journey and highlight correlations between activities and flare-ups, making the path to management feel much clearer and manageable.

Helpful Apps for Arthritis Management

There are many mobile apps designed specifically to help individuals manage their arthritis effectively.

These apps offer a wide variety of features, such as tracking symptoms, recording medication schedules, and providing educational resources. As someone who has navigated the challenges of arthritis, I've found these tools to be incredibly supportive. For instance, some apps allow you to input daily pain levels, which helps in identifying patterns and triggers. By maintaining a detailed log of your physical condition, you can engage in more informed conversations with your healthcare providers. Additionally, many apps come equipped with reminders for medication and hydration, encouraging you to stay on top of your regimen, which is crucial for managing arthritis.

Technology can be a powerful ally in your journey towards better health. Utilizing these apps not only assists with symptom tracking but also empowers you to educate yourself about your condition. Many of them provide articles and tips on managing pain, nutrition advice, and ways to improve mobility, all tailored to your specific needs as an arthritis warrior. Engaging with these resources can be both motivating and enlightening, reminding you that you are not alone in your battle. Embracing this technology can transform the way you view your condition, allowing you to take control of your health with the knowledge and insights these apps offer.

A practical tip to enhance your experience with these apps is to commit to daily check-ins. Whether it's in the morning with a quick session to log your symptoms or in the evening to review your day, consistency is key. Over time, you'll uncover valuable insights into your health patterns, making it easier to advocate for yourself and adjust your treatment as needed. Remember, the goal is to harness these technological tools to live not just with arthritis, but to thrive despite it.

Staying Connected through Technology

Technology serves as a vital bridge for maintaining connections with loved ones, especially for those facing the challenges of arthritis. It allows us to stay in touch, share moments, and support each other even when mobility becomes an issue. I remember the days when a simple phone call was a lifeline, but now we have so many more options. Video calls, messaging apps, and social networks can bring a sense of closeness that might feel lost when physical distance or pain separates us. For instance, being able to see my family's faces during a video chat always brightens my day and reassures me that I am not alone in my struggles.

These tools help to combat the feelings of isolation that can creep in when physical meetings aren't possible. By sending a quick text or sharing a photo through an app, I create a connection that feels alive. It's encouraging to know that with just a few taps on my screen, I can reach out and remind someone I care about them. This connection can be crucial for managing the emotional pain that sometimes accompanies arthritis, reinforcing the feeling that we are part of a caring community. The more we communicate, the more we combat loneliness, proving that love truly knows no boundaries, even those imposed by our health.

For those of us living with arthritis, the physical limitations can heighten feelings of isolation, making it challenging to engage in activities we once enjoyed. Yet, communication tools have become a lifeline, helping to bridge the gap created by discomfort and fatigue. With arthritis affecting our mobility and strength, arranging in-person gatherings can be daunting. Thankfully, platforms like social media and video conferencing offer flexible alternatives. I often find solace in participating in online support groups where experiences and encouragement are shared among those who truly understand what it's like.

Engaging in conversations through these digital platforms allows for a sense of belonging without the need for extensive physical effort. Friends and family can join in at a time that suits them, making it easier to maintain those crucial connections. I have discovered that sharing my feelings about living with arthritis sparks conversations that can lead to deeper support and understanding. In this way, technology becomes not just a communication tool, but also a source of community and empowerment. It reminds us that while we may face challenges, we can still reach out and be reached, reinforcing the bonds that matter most. Utilizing these tools can transform our experiences, allowing us to thrive socially, despite the physical limitations we endure.

Try setting up regular virtual hangouts or check-ins with loved ones. Making that effort can greatly enhance your emotional health and remind you that you're not alone in your journey.

Chapter 16: Mobility Aids

Types of Mobility Aids

Arthritis can be a daunting challenge, hindering basic movements and making everyday tasks feel insurmountable. Luckily, a range of mobility aids is available, designed to help individuals regain independence and confidence. From canes and walkers to scooters and specialized chairs, each aid serves a distinct purpose, catering specifically to the unique needs of arthritis sufferers. Understanding the options can help you choose the right aid for your situation and daily activities. I've personally navigated this journey, experiencing firsthand how a simple device can transform the way I approach my day. Mobility aids are more than just tools; they are life-changing companions on the path toward maintaining an active and fulfilling life despite the limitations arthritis can impose.

Each type of mobility aid comes with its own set of benefits, tailored to different levels of mobility and personal preferences. For instance, a cane can be an excellent choice for those who need a little extra support while walking but are still fairly mobile. Canes not only help to stabilize your posture but also reduce strain on the joints, enabling smoother movement. Walkers, on the other hand, offer additional support and balance, making them ideal for individuals who require more stability while walking. They can distribute weight more evenly, alleviating pressure on painful joints. As I transitioned from using a cane to a walker, I felt an incredible sense of security, allowing me to venture further outside my home without fear of falling.

If mobility becomes significantly restricted, powered mobility scooters and electric wheelchairs can offer a dose of freedom. These devices allow for effortless navigation of both indoor and outdoor spaces, and they empower individuals to participate in social activities without feeling hindered by their condition. I remember the first time I tried a scooter at a family gathering; the exhilaration of being able to join conversations and navigate through the crowd was genuinely uplifting. Specialized chairs can also play a vital role in enhancing comfort during resting periods. They are designed to provide maximum support for the back and joints, making it easier to get up and down when required. It's important to explore these aids with an open mind and recognize that they are not signifiers of weakness; rather, they are wonderful companions that facilitate a more independent and enjoyable lifestyle. When considering mobility aids, keep in mind that starting small and building your confidence can lead to a more empowered approach to managing arthritis in your life. Exploring options and trying different aids can open up possibilities you never thought possible.

Choosing the Right Aid for Your Needs

Finding the right mobility aid can feel overwhelming, especially when each option seems tailored to someone else's needs. Understanding that your mobility aid should reflect your individual requirements is essential. Consider how often you will use it, the types of activities you enjoy, and the spaces you frequently navigate. Are you mostly indoor-bound, or do you venture outside often? You might need a cane for quick trips or a walker for support during longer outings. Some aids are more stable, while others are lightweight and easy to carry. Whether you choose a scooter, a wheelchair, or a simple walking aid, remember that it should enhance your daily life, not hinder it. Take your time exploring different options, and don't hesitate to seek advice from healthcare professionals who understand your unique situation. What works best for one person may not be right for you, and that's okay; this journey is about what makes you feel secure and free.

Assessing your mobility needs thoroughly means taking a moment to reflect on your day-to-day life. Think about what challenges you face while moving. Do you find it hard to stand for long periods? Do you sometimes feel fatigued after short walks? It's also helpful to consider your surroundings. Are there stairs, uneven surfaces, or narrow doorways that could make mobility difficult? Observation of your body's signals is crucial. Perhaps you've noticed that walking distances leave you breathing heavily, or you struggle with balance, reflecting these experiences can guide you in making informed choices. Talk with family members or friends who understand your situation; their insights might highlight things you overlook. The goal is to enhance your independence and ensure you feel confident moving around your home and community. Don't rush this process; understanding your mobility needs is about kindness to yourself.

Prioritize comfort, safety, and ease of use as you explore your options. It can be helpful to try out various mobility aids in store settings or through rental programs. This hands-on experience can make the selection process less daunting and more tailored to your life. Don't shy away from asking for specific features that matter to you, like lightweight designs, easy adjustments, or comfortable grips. Remember, the right mobility aid is not merely a tool; it's a companion that will support you in living life to the fullest. While exploring these options, keep in mind that patience is key. Celebrate the small victories along the way, whether it's a successful test-run of a new device or simply a good conversation with someone who understands what you're going through. Ultimately, the right choice will resonate with your personal needs and empower you to engage with the world around you more fully.

Using Aids in Different Areas of the Home

Mobility aids can make a significant difference in how we navigate our homes, especially when living with a condition that affects movement. Each room in your home may present unique challenges, but understanding how to effectively use aids can empower you. In the living room, for instance, ensuring that your walker or cane is at your side can avoid unnecessary strain. If you use a wheelchair, clearing space to maneuver is critical. When you're sitting down, consider the height of your seating. Using cushions might help you rise easily and safely. Always ensure that pathways are clear, and if you have furniture that can be rearranged, do not hesitate to make those adjustments. This small change can significantly enhance your freedom of movement, making your home feel more yours.

When it comes to optimizing the use of aids, comfort and safety should always guide your choices. Beyond just finding the right equipment, think about how you can create an environment that supports your needs.

For your bathroom, non-slip mats can help prevent falls, and installing grab bars near the shower or bathtub can provide extra stability. In the kitchen, using a shower chair can allow you to rest while washing, preserving your energy for other activities. Adjustments like lowering shelf heights or using a reacher tool can prevent unnecessary stretching and lifting, ensuring safety. Listen to your body and make these improvements because the goal is to enhance your independence while feeling secure in your surroundings.

Taking the time to assess your home and your needs leads to better choices in mobility aids, and remember to involve family and friends in these discussions. They can provide valuable support, helping you create an environment that works for you. Share your thoughts about what aids enhance your daily life, and don't hesitate to ask for assistance when needed. The more proactive you are in adapting your home, the more poised you will feel in controlling your space. Even simple changes can boost your confidence immensely. A useful tip is to keep a small journal of what works for you and what doesn't as you navigate different areas of your home; this can help you refine your approach over time.

Maintaining Mobility Aids

Maintaining mobility aids is essential for ensuring they function effectively when you need them most. Regular cleaning is a fundamental practice that cannot be overlooked. Dust, dirt, and grime can accumulate over time, leading to deterioration. Depending on the type of aid—whether it's a walker, wheelchair, or crutches—most can be easily cleaned with a damp cloth and mild soap. For wheelchairs, it's important to focus on the wheels and undercarriage, where debris often hides. Regularly check for any signs of wear or damage, such as fraying straps, rust, or cracks. If you notice any issues, it's vital to address them immediately, as neglecting repairs can lead to bigger problems down the line.

Another key practice is to ensure the moving parts, like wheels and hinges, are well-lubricated. This can help prevent squeaks and will make sure your mobility aid operates smoothly. Adjustments to straps or height settings should also be checked periodically, as they can shift with use. When it comes to storage, choose a dry, cool spot, away from direct sunlight and excessive humidity. Protect your mobility aid from extreme temperatures, which can warp or degrade materials over time. By taking these simple steps for upkeep, you can foster a reliable relationship with your mobility aid that empowers your daily life.

The longevity of your mobility aids is partly determined by how well you take care of them. Regular inspections are a vital part of this process. For wheelchairs, check the tires for wear and ensure they are inflated to the proper pressure. If you are using a cane or walker, make sure the rubber tips are intact and free from cracks. These seemingly minor details can prevent accidents and provide stability when you're on the move. Additionally, consider the terrain you navigate regularly. If you often find yourself in rough or uneven environments, investing in specialized tires or cushions can significantly enhance the performance and durability of your mobility aids.

Consider keeping a log or diary of maintenance checks. Jotting down what you inspect, when you clean, and when repairs are made can help you spot patterns and anticipate future maintenance needs. It can also offer you peace of mind, knowing that you're being proactive. Remember, your mobility aids are not just tools; they are extensions of your body, helping you regain independence. By treating them with care and respect, you're not only prolonging their life but also enhancing your own quality of life. A practical tip to remember is to invest in a good repair kit tailored for your mobility device. Having basic tools and replacement parts on hand can make addressing minor issues less cumbersome.

Alternative Mobility Solutions

Many people often find themselves facing the challenge of mobility, whether due to physical limitations, age, or unexpected situations. Exploring alternative solutions can illuminate a path beyond traditional aids like wheelchairs and canes. These aids, though valuable, don't always fit the rich tapestry of individual experiences. It's about thinking outside the box, about mobility not just as a means to move but as a gateway to experience life fully. Innovations such as adaptive bicycles, electric scooters, or even community-based ridesharing options present unique ways to enhance mobility. Technologies like smart walking aids and exoskeletons can empower individuals with new possibilities that resonate with their specific needs and lifestyle. Understanding that mobility challenges do not define one's abilities is the first step toward embracing these alternatives.

Encouraging innovative concepts and adaptations requires us to cultivate an open mindset. Every individual's journey is unique, and creative solutions might lie in unexpected areas. Consider engaging with local community groups that focus on mobility challenges; they often have resources and ideas that emerge not only from technological advancements but also from shared experiences. Think about how easy it could be to collaborate with local businesses, artists, or inventors to design customized tools that suit personal needs. There is tremendous power in experimentation and adaptation. Your idea could lead to a breakthrough that not only transforms your mobility but inspires others on similar journeys. Remember, innovation often starts from empathy and understanding—recognizing what others have experienced can guide you toward impactful solutions.

As you explore these possibilities, don't hesitate to communicate openly about your needs. Sharing your experience not only brings awareness but can spark conversations that inspire others to consider and develop alternative mobility solutions. You have the ability to create change, whether through blogging, participating in forums, or even starting community projects. Every voice counts, and together, we can drive a movement that celebrates mobility in all its forms. A practical step to begin with is to jot down your personal mobility experiences, challenges, and ideas. This reflection can serve as a vital tool, guiding you as you navigate through options and pave the way toward a future filled with possibilities.

Chapter 17: Community Resources

Local Support Groups

Joining local support groups can significantly impact our lives. Sharing our experiences with others who understand our struggles can be incredibly comforting. In these gatherings, there's a unique sense of freedom as we open up, revealing thoughts and feelings we often keep bottled up. When we talk about our challenges, we not only find empathy but also encouragement from those who truly get it. Their stories resonate with us, reminding us we are not alone in our thirst for understanding and connection. The camaraderie found in these groups fosters a sense of community that can motivate us to keep pressing forward, even when the path gets tough.

Community support plays a crucial role in enhancing our coping strategies. When we are surrounded by people who have faced similar challenges, we can learn from their experiences. We discover new ways to handle our emotions, strategies to manage our daily lives, and techniques to uplift our spirits. The group environment encourages open discussions about feelings and practical coping methods, which can help us rethink our own approaches. As we share tips and personal anecdotes, we build a toolkit of resources to draw on when things get overwhelming. This shared knowledge becomes powerful, turning our individual struggles into collective strength.

Being part of a support group isn't just about receiving help; it's also about giving it. When we support others, we reinforce our own healing. It's empowering to see how our experiences can inspire someone else to persevere. This dual dynamic of sharing and supporting fosters an atmosphere of hope and resilience. It reminds us that while our journeys may feel solitary at times, there exists a network of individuals who walk similar paths, making the journey a little less daunting. Consider seeking out a local support group. Even just attending once can spark new ideas and connections that enrich your life beyond measure.

Therapeutic Services Available

Therapeutic services for individuals dealing with arthritis can provide a valuable source of support and relief. Arthritis can be a relentless companion, affecting daily life and limiting mobility. Thankfully, a variety of therapeutic options are accessible to help manage the pain and improve the quality of life. Physical therapy is one such service that focuses on individualized exercises and stretches tailored to enhance joint function and reduce discomfort. A skilled therapist can work with you to develop a personalized plan that helps strengthen muscles around the affected joints, improve flexibility, and enhance overall movement. Occupational therapy also plays a pivotal role by teaching individuals how to adapt daily activities to maintain independence while minimizing strain on the joints. Integrating assistive devices and modifying workspaces can significantly reduce stress on arthritic joints.

In addition to these traditional therapies, alternative modalities such as acupuncture and massage therapy can be incredibly beneficial. Acupuncture, which involves inserting thin needles at specific points, has been reported to relieve pain and reduce inflammation for many individuals. On the other hand, massage therapy can promote relaxation and alleviate tension in sore muscles, offering a heightened sense of well-being. Exploring these various therapeutic approaches can empower you to take control of your arthritis management. It might take some experimentation to find what resonates best with you, but engaging with different therapies can lead to surprising improvements in your comfort and mobility.

Take the time to research and connect with local practitioners or health centers that specialize in arthritis care. Many communities offer support groups where you can share experiences and gain insights into what has worked for others on a similar journey. Remember that your body is unique, and while one method might work wonders for someone else, discovering your perfect combination of therapies can take time. Stay open-minded, and don't shy away from asking questions or voicing concerns with your healthcare providers. They are there to guide and support you. Make it a priority to seek out these services; a more comfortable, active lifestyle is within your reach. Consider starting a simple daily routine of gentle exercises, as this can lay a solid foundation for further therapeutic interventions.

Healthcare Providers for Arthritis

Finding healthcare providers who specialize in arthritis care can feel overwhelming. Most likely, you want someone who understands not just the technical aspects of the disease, but also how it affects your daily life. Rheumatologists are perhaps your primary go-to specialists. These doctors focus on diagnosing and treating arthritis and related conditions. They have the skills to manage your treatment plan, adjusting medications to find that delicate balance between effectiveness and minimizing side effects. However, the journey doesn't end there. Physical therapists are equally essential in your support system. They can design personalized exercise programs that help you maintain mobility and reduce pain. Occupational therapists can introduce adaptive tools and strategies that make daily tasks easier, giving you back some independence. When cradled in the right network, these professionals work collaboratively to provide comprehensive care tailored to your specific circumstances.

The beauty of interdisciplinary care cannot be overstated when managing arthritis. It's not just about consulting multiple providers; it's about their ability to communicate and coordinate effectively. Imagine sitting at a round table, where your rheumatologist, physical therapist, and occupational therapist come together to discuss your progress. This team approach can lead to a more nuanced understanding of how various aspects of your life interact with your condition. For example, what your physical therapist suggests can greatly influence the medication adjustments your rheumatologist might consider. Likewise, an occupational therapist's insights can shed light on how to incorporate effective exercises into your routine. As they work together, you become an integral part of the conversation, not just a bystander, which can help you feel more empowered in your treatment.

Establishing strong communication with your healthcare providers can significantly enhance your overall management of arthritis. Don't hesitate to ask questions or express concerns. The more open the dialogue, the better your care can be adapted to fit your needs. As a practical tip, consider preparing a list of your symptoms, any changes you notice, and questions before your appointments. This can help ensure that your healthcare providers address all your concerns, giving you a clearer path in your journey toward managing arthritis. Staying engaged with each member of your care team fosters a sense of community and support that can be incredibly motivating on the road to wellness.

Educational Workshops and Seminars

Attending workshops to learn more about arthritis and its management can profoundly impact your life. Knowledge is a powerful tool when dealing with a condition that often feels overwhelming. These workshops provide a safe space for you to share your experiences, hear others' stories, and learn from healthcare professionals who truly understand arthritis. Engaging with experts allows you to ask questions and gain insights that might otherwise take years to accumulate. You discover practical strategies for managing pain, improving mobility, and enhancing your overall quality of life. This shared journey fosters a sense of community, reminding you that you are not alone in this battle. Each workshop opens doors to understanding your condition better, helping you regain a sense of control over your health.

Education goes beyond just understanding a diagnosis; it's about skills development and empowerment. Workshops often focus on teaching you essential skills such as exercise techniques tailored for arthritis, stress management strategies, and dietary advice that can ease inflammation. They equip you with the knowledge to advocate for yourself in medical settings, ensuring you make informed decisions about your treatment options. Participating in these events also provides a chance to learn new coping mechanisms that can be seamlessly integrated into your daily life. Whether it's through hands-on activities or interactive discussions, each session sparks motivation and equips you with tools to live more fully. It's about unlocking your potential and discovering new ways to thrive despite the challenges that arthritis presents.

Engaging in workshops fosters personal connections, and sharing experiences with others can alleviate feelings of isolation. Each conversation held during these sessions can inspire hope and ignite the desire for a more fulfilling life while managing arthritis. One practical tip is to seek out both local workshops and online webinars, as these options cater to different levels of comfort and accessibility. Find a group that resonates with you; sometimes, it only takes one conversation to change your perspective and set you on a new path toward better health.

Advocacy and Awareness Programs

Understanding the importance of advocacy in raising awareness about arthritis is essential for all of us who live with this condition. The journey of dealing with arthritis can feel isolating, but together, we can make our voices heard. Advocacy plays a crucial role in educating others, including friends, family, and the broader community, about what arthritis truly means. By sharing our personal stories and challenges, we help break down stereotypes and misconceptions that surround this condition. This isn't just about sharing facts; it's about fostering empathy and understanding. When we advocate for arthritis awareness, we are not merely highlighting a medical issue; we are humanizing it. It brings to light the daily struggles we face, encouraging people to see us not just as patients, but as individuals with hopes, dreams, and real-life battles. Through advocacy, we can inspire changes in policies and practices that ultimately benefit all who are affected.

Encouragement to participate in or support awareness initiatives can make a tremendous difference. It's inspiring to see how collective efforts can elevate the conversation around arthritis. Whether you choose to participate in local events, join online communities, or support advocacy organizations, your involvement is valuable. Sharing your experience, no matter how small it may seem, can have a ripple effect. It encourages others to speak up, participate, and educate those around them. You can inspire someone else who might feel alone or overwhelmed, showing them that they are part of a larger community that truly cares. Moreover, supporting awareness initiatives not only raises attention but also fosters hope. By coming together, we can influence research, drive funding, and advocate for better treatments that could enhance our quality of life. Every little step counts, and by taking part in these initiatives, you become a beacon of hope for others living with arthritis.

One practical tip to enhance your advocacy efforts is to share your story on social media. Platforms like Facebook, Instagram, and Twitter offer a space to connect with others and spread awareness like wildfire. Use your words, photos, or videos to make it personal. Talk about your daily life with arthritis, the challenges you face, or even the small victories that bring you joy. Make it relatable—people are more likely to engage with real-life stories. This simple act can open the door for conversations, spark curiosity, and draw others into the fold of understanding and empathy. Remember, your voice matters, and sharing it can help create the change we all seek.

Chapter 18: Family Involvement

Educating Family Members

Understanding arthritis is a journey that requires the involvement of the entire family. When family members grasp the nature of this condition and the unique challenges it presents, they can become instrumental in offering support. Sharing my experience, it was enlightening to see how my struggles with arthritis manifested in various daily tasks like cooking, cleaning, or even just getting out of bed. It wasn't just about the pain in my joints; it had ripple effects on my mood, my energy, and my ability to participate in family life. With educating my loved ones, I emphasized that it wasn't just me trapped in this cycle, but that we were in it together. In doing so, they learned to empathize with my restrictions and understand that some days would be harder than others. This awareness helped in creating more meaningful conversations about expectations for family outings or daily chores, leading to a greater understanding of what it meant to live with arthritis.

Cultivating a supportive and understanding home environment is paramount when living with arthritis. It requires open lines of communication, patience, and a willingness to adapt. For instance, we started discussing my limitations openly, like when my joints flared up, communication became crucial in preventing misunderstandings. The days I could join in family activities or prepare dinner were shared celebratory moments. When those days were limited, I appreciated their help more than I could express.

This mutual understanding reassured me that I wasn't a burden but rather a part of a team willing to adjust for the sake of each other's well-being. Activities were organized around my capabilities, fostering not just patience but also a stronger bond among family members, establishing a vibrant atmosphere of encouragement that nurtured emotional connection.

Ultimately, it's about creating a culture within the family where empathy flourishes. Encouraging family members to ask questions about my condition or share resources they've found relevant can spark discussions leading to deeper understanding. Simple actions, like preparing meals that require fewer ingredients or volunteering to help with housework or errands on particularly tough days, go a long way. Each small step turns into a significant gesture of love and consideration, laying a solid foundation that helps everyone navigate the complexities of living with arthritis together. Keeping the lines of communication open transforms moments of frustration into opportunities for connection and support, making every member feel valued and understood.

Encouraging Participation

Encouraging family members to actively participate in your care can be a transformative experience for everyone involved. It often starts with open and honest communication about your needs and preferences. Share your feelings about how their support would make a difference in your journey. When family members understand the impact of their involvement, they may feel more compelled to step in and offer help. Engaging them in conversations about your care can also foster a deeper emotional connection, allowing them to realize that your journey is a shared experience. Consider setting aside a time each week for family discussions about your progress and any adjustments needed in your care plan. These meetings can become a focal point for collaboration, enabling them to voice their thoughts and concerns while feeling a part of the process.

Creating a culture of collaboration and support within your family involves nurturing an environment where everyone feels valued and heard. Encouragement should flow freely both ways; express gratitude for the small things they do, and invite them to encourage each other as well. Highlighting the importance of teamwork can create a sense of unity. Foster an atmosphere where family members can voice their feelings without judgment. When your loved ones feel safe to share their thoughts, they are more likely to engage. You can consider scheduling regular family activities unrelated to care, which can strengthen bonds and minimize any focus on illness or challenges. These occasions serve as a reminder of the joy and love that exist within your family, reinforcing the idea that you are all in this together, supporting one another through thick and thin.

Remember that involving family members in your care involves patience and commitment. Encourage them to take ownership of certain aspects, whether it's managing appointments or helping with daily tasks. This not only lightens your burden but also empowers them. They may have insights or solutions that you haven't considered. Use gentle nudges to invite participation; everyone's contribution, no matter how small, counts. Consider creating a shared calendar or a group chat to coordinate efforts and share updates to maintain momentum. This ensures that everyone is on the same page and feels an integral part of your care journey.

Creating a Supportive Home Environment

Designing a family environment that fosters support and understanding involves being intentional with our space and interactions. It's about creating a sanctuary where everyone feels safe to express themselves without fear of judgment. Consider the layout of your home; open spaces can encourage togetherness, while cozy nooks can offer a retreat for individuals to recharge. Elements like family photos, shared accomplishments, or even art created by your children can create a visual narrative that reminds everyone of their shared experiences and love. Simple acts, like dedicating a regular family night or creating a communal space for shared projects, can strengthen bonds. When family members feel the environment is a reflection of their values and memories, they are more likely to cherish and maintain that supportive atmosphere.

The importance of communication and shared goals cannot be overstated in fostering a supportive home. Engaging in regular family discussions to articulate dreams, aspirations, and even everyday frustrations helps create a sense of belonging. It's essential that every member feels their voice matters, fostering an inclusive atmosphere. Setting shared goals, whether they are related to personal growth, family trips, or collective projects, fosters teamwork and strengthens unity. These goals act as a beacon, guiding everyone towards common aspirations while celebrating individual contributions. When we communicate openly and encourage each other's dreams, we build a foundation of trust and respect which is vital in the journey towards a supportive living space.

As you reflect on your family environment, consider establishing a "family mission statement" together. This can encapsulate your shared values and goals, serving as a constant reminder of your commitment to one another. Taking the time to articulate what is important to each of you strengthens the understanding that a loving, supportive home doesn't just happen; it is nurtured through consistent effort and communication.

Family Activities That Promote Mobility

Engaging in activities that promote mobility within the family can be both fun and beneficial for everyone involved. Simple outings like family walks in the park can transform into an opportunity for exercise and bonding. As we stroll through nature, watching the leaves rustle and feeling the sun on our faces, conversations naturally flow. This creates not just a healthy habit, but also memorable moments that strengthen our relationships. Another great idea is biking together. Whether it's cycling at a nearby trail or just around the neighborhood, biking is a fantastic way to boost heart rates and enjoy each other's company. The excitement of racing each other to a finish line or stopping to take pictures along the way can make the activity enjoyable for all ages. Even playful activities at home, such as dance-offs in the living room, can be surprisingly effective. These moments not only get everyone moving but also allow for laughter and light-hearted competition.

Encouraging shared experiences is essential for enhancing family bonds. When we partake in activities together, we build lasting memories that we can cherish for years to come. Cooking meals as a family can be surprisingly effective in bringing everyone closer. Choosing a recipe that involves some movement—like kneading dough or chopping vegetables—can create an engaging environment. Additionally, sharing stories and traditions while preparing food fosters a sense of belonging. Team sports, such as basketball or soccer, can also strengthen these connections. Playing as a team encourages collaboration and teamwork, reinforcing the idea that we are all striving towards a common goal. Such moments of working together—be it through a friendly game or community service, like a family cleanup day—help us understand the importance of togetherness, resilience, and support.

Remember, even small gestures can create a significant impact. Plan regular family activity nights dedicated to engaging in any mobility-promoting activities, no matter how simple. Designate one evening a week to try out something new or revisit a favorite pastime. It could be a walk, a game of tag, or even a fun exercise video that everyone enjoys. The key is to create consistency and integration of movement into family life, allowing it to become a core part of your routine. By doing so, not only will you enhance your family's overall health, but you will also weave a tapestry of shared experiences that bind your family closer together.

Communication and Understanding

Open communication can often feel like a lifeline when facing the challenges of arthritis. Sharing feelings with loved ones about the daily struggles, whether related to pain, fatigue, or the limitations of movement, creates an environment where support and understanding can thrive. When I began talking openly about my experiences, I realized how many people were coping with similar issues. Simply voicing my thoughts about what I was feeling helped to diminish some of the isolation that often accompanies chronic illness. Those conversations not only clarified my needs and limits but also helped my family and friends understand how they could better support me. It was empowering to discuss openly not only the pain but also the good days when I felt more in control, reinforcing the fact that I am more than my condition.

Mutual understanding plays a crucial role in developing effective coping strategies. In my journey with arthritis, I found that when I expressed my struggles and fears, it opened the door to deeper conversations, where others could share their perspectives and support. This exchange built a bridge of compassion and empathy, which made us all feel more connected. Knowing that family and friends were aware of my pain on good days and bad days allowed us to navigate activities together, reducing tension and enhancing experiences. In moments when I felt overwhelmed, my loved ones could offer a comforting presence because I had taken the time to explain what I was going through. This created a safe space for use to discuss adjustments that needed to be made and strategize on how to handle particular situations, whether that meant adjusting plans or simply taking a break when necessary. Through this collaborative approach, I began to realize that adapting to my condition didn't mean sacrificing joy or connection; instead, it led to a more enriching experience filled with understanding and love.

In your own journey, consider taking small steps toward open dialogue. Find a quiet moment to share your feelings or thoughts about arthritis with someone close to you. Those simple conversations can pave the way for mutual understanding and foster a supportive environment, making a significant difference in how you navigate your daily challenges.

Chapter 19: Nutrition and Diet

Food Choices that Impact Arthritis

Food can play a crucial role in managing arthritis, touching both our bodies and our emotions. Certain types of foods can either ease the pain and inflammation or exacerbate the symptoms we face. For example, omega-3 fatty acids found in fatty fish like salmon and sardines can help reduce joint inflammation. The power of fruits and vegetables cannot be overstated either; they are packed with antioxidants and anti-inflammatory compounds. Berries, in particular, like blueberries and strawberries, can be your allies in the fight against inflammation. On the flip side, processed foods and those high in sugar can be detrimental. They may worsen inflammation and trigger more severe arthritis symptoms. Foods like white bread, fried items, and snacks loaded with refined sugars can provoke flares and irritate your joints. Becoming more aware of what we consume can significantly influence how we feel daily.

Making informed dietary choices isn't just about avoiding certain foods; it's about embracing those that nurture our bodies and promote better joint health. I can assure you that transitioning to a healthier diet doesn't have to be overwhelming. Start by incorporating one or two new anti-inflammatory foods into your meals each week. Maybe add some leafy greens like spinach or kale to your daily salad or enjoy a handful of nuts as a snack. It's about making incremental changes that serve your well-being.

Listen to your body. Notice how certain foods make you feel and adjust accordingly. This personal journey towards better food choices is empowering. It allows you to reclaim some control over your arthritis, turning the focus towards how each bite can move you closer to feeling good. Your relationship with food can become a positive part of managing arthritis, providing both nourishment and comfort.

Practical tips can make a significant difference in your journey. Keep a food journal where you note what you eat and how it affects your arthritis symptoms. This simple step can help you find patterns and identify which foods are your friends and which ones can be triggers. Ultimately, you have the power to shape your dietary landscape in a way that supports both your body and your spirit.

Meal Planning for Joint Health

When it comes to meal planning that emphasizes anti-inflammatory ingredients, the focus should be on whole, nutrient-dense foods. Incorporating a rainbow of fruits and vegetables is a great starting point, as they are rich in antioxidants that can help reduce inflammation. I've found that leafy greens, such as kale and spinach, not only add vital nutrients but also provide a satisfying texture to meals. Adding fatty fish, like salmon or mackerel, brings in omega-3 fatty acids, known for their ability to lower inflammation and pain associated with arthritis. Another helpful ingredient is turmeric. This vibrant spice, with its active compound curcumin, offers powerful anti-inflammatory benefits. A simple way to incorporate it is by adding it to soups, stews, or even smoothies. Moreover, whole grains like quinoa and brown rice can be fantastic sources of fiber, which can help reduce inflammation and support overall health. Pay attention to your sources of protein as well; beans and legumes are not only delicious but also low in saturated fat, making them a great choice for joint health.

Thinking about the kinds of meals that are both nutritious and arthritis-friendly can be quite empowering. I've learned that hearty soups and stews can be a comforting option. They can be packed with a variety of vegetables and lean proteins, simmered to perfection with anti-inflammatory spices. For instance, a chickpea and vegetable stew can be both filling and incredibly nutritious. Another fantastic meal idea is a colorful salad topped with grilled salmon, avocado, and a drizzle of olive oil and lemon juice, which combine healthy fats with fresh ingredients to nourish your joints. Stir-fries are also a wonderful choice; they allow you to include various vegetables like bell peppers and broccoli, along with lean protein like chicken or tofu. These meals can be made quickly and customized with whatever ingredients you have on hand. Snacks can also be a part of this plan, so considering things like nuts, seeds, or hummus with carrot sticks can keep your energy levels stable while supporting joint health.

Transitioning to meals that prioritize joint health may require some adjustments, but even small steps can lead to significant benefits. Keeping a meal plan that focuses on anti-inflammatory foods doesn't mean sacrificing taste or variety. Instead, it's about creating a lifestyle that embraces cooking and enjoying meals made from scratch. Finding joy in preparing foods that help you feel better can be motivating, and even involving family or friends in the process can turn cooking into a fun social activity. Remember, it's about balance. Give yourself permission to enjoy your favorite foods on occasion. This approach helps create a sustainable habit that supports not only your joint health but your overall well-being, turning meal planning into an opportunity for nourishment, creativity, and connection.

Supplements to Consider

Living with arthritis can feel like an endless battle, but there are supplements that might help ease some of the discomfort. Many individuals dealing with arthritis have found potential relief in anti-inflammatory supplements. Omega-3 fatty acids, commonly found in fish oil, have gained attention for their ability to reduce joint stiffness and inflammation. Curcumin, the active compound in turmeric, is another supplement that has shown promise. It is noted for its anti-inflammatory properties and may even help improve overall joint function. Additionally, glucosamine and chondroitin sulfate are often mentioned in discussions about joint health. These substances could potentially aid in rebuilding cartilage and alleviating pain associated with osteoarthritis. However, it is essential to remember that everyone's body is unique, and what works for one person might not work for another.

Before making any changes to your supplement routine, it is crucial to consult with a healthcare provider. They can offer personalized advice based on your health history and current medications, ensuring that any supplements you consider won't interact adversely with your existing treatments. It is understandable to seek out alternatives that may help with pain management, but healthcare professionals can guide you through the options, emphasizing safe usage and appropriate dosages. Engaging in a conversation with your provider can empower you to make informed decisions tailored specifically to your needs, which is vital on the journey of managing arthritis.

Finding the right approach might take some time, but being proactive about exploring options can bring hope. Keeping a journal of your symptoms and any supplements you choose can offer valuable insights over time. This practice allows you to track what helps and what doesn't, leading to more productive discussions with your healthcare provider. Remember, you are not alone in this journey, and taking these steps could help you discover more effective ways to manage your arthritis.

Hydration and Its Importance

Staying well-hydrated is crucial for our overall health and the smooth function of our joints. Many people underestimate how important water is for energy levels, digestion, and even mood. During my journey of wellness, I've realized that hydration is one of the simplest yet most profound ways to care for my body. When I prioritize drinking enough water, I notice a significant decrease in fatigue and joint stiffness. My body feels more vibrant, and I'm able to move with ease during workouts and daily activities. Those moments when I've let my fluid intake slide have taught me that our joints, which often bear the brunt of our daily movements, rely on water for lubrication. Proper hydration helps to cushion joints and reduces the likelihood of pain or discomfort. It is a fundamental aspect of maintaining an active lifestyle, supporting not only physical health but emotional well-being too.

To ensure adequate hydration throughout the day, I've developed a few strategies that work for me, and I believe they can benefit others as well. One effective method is to carry a water bottle everywhere I go. It serves as a constant reminder to drink water regularly and keeps hydration top of mind. Setting specific hydration goals also helps; for instance, I aim to drink a glass of water before each meal and at least one after every workout. This practice has turned drinking water into a natural part of my routine. Adding flavor to my water, like slices of lemon or cucumber, has made it more enjoyable, encouraging me to drink even more. Finally, I pay attention to my body's signals; whenever I feel fatigue creeping in, I shift my focus to my water intake, often finding that a refreshing drink can re-energize me and support my joints at the same time. Remembering that hydration can affect our mood and performance is a powerful motivator to keep that water flowing.

One practical tip to boost your hydration is to establish a water-drinking cue, like having a sip every time you check your phone or complete a task. This way, you create a habit that blends seamlessly into your daily life. Make it fun and stay aware; staying hydrated is your ally for a healthier and more active lifestyle.

Cooking Methods that Reduce Inflammation

Understanding how the way we cook can influence our health is crucial, especially when it comes to managing inflammation. There are several cooking methods that can actually help minimize inflammatory responses in the body. For instance, steaming vegetables preserves their nutrients better than boiling or frying, which can deplete vitamins and minerals. Grilling and roasting meats are also effective since they allow excess fats to drip away, reducing the consumption of potentially harmful saturated fats. When it comes to plant-based meals, partaking in methods like sautéing using healthy oils, such as olive oil or avocado oil, can enhance the absorption of beneficial nutrients while adding a rich flavor. Additionally, incorporating slow cooking or pressure cooking not only tenderizes tough meats but also retains moisture and nutrients, providing hearty meals full of flavors and health benefits. These methods can help create dishes that are both satisfying and supportive of our wellbeing.

Healthy cooking practices are essential in supporting overall wellness and alleviating symptoms associated with inflammation. When I switched to preparing meals in a way that prioritizes health, I found that not only did my energy levels improve, but so did my mood. Emphasizing whole foods in my cooking made a world of difference; fresh fruits, vegetables, whole grains, and lean proteins became my staples. One practical approach is to experiment with herbs and spices known for their anti-inflammatory properties, such as turmeric, ginger, and cinnamon. Adding these to dishes not only boosts their flavor but also enhances their health benefits. Opting for fresh ingredients and avoiding processed foods reduced my intake of additives that can exacerbate inflammation. It's also rewarding to dedicate time to meal prep; I've learned that preparing meals in advance not only saves me time during the week but also ensures that I have healthy options readily available, steering me away from unhealthy choices when I'm busy.

When you embrace cooking as a means to nourish your body, every meal becomes an opportunity for healing. A simple but powerful practice is to always cook with intention; this means being mindful of ingredients and how they interact to promote health. When stirring up a pot of soup or tossing a salad, consider the colors and richness of each ingredient. Each vibrant color signifies different nutrients and benefits. Be creative and enjoy the process, as cooking can be therapeutic. Remember, it's not just about what you eat, but how you prepare it. By focusing on these methods and practices, one can transform their approach to food and find relief from inflammation.

Chapter 20: Exercise and Movement

The Importance of Regular Movement

Regular movement plays a crucial role in managing arthritis symptoms. When I first started experiencing arthritis, I struggled with stiffness, pain, and fatigue. Simple movements felt daunting, and I often avoided them altogether. However, I learned that maintaining an active lifestyle is essential for joint health. Moving helps lubricate the joints, reduces stiffness, and improves circulation, making everyday activities more manageable. There were days when the thought of getting up to stretch felt overwhelming, but I've discovered that even gentle movements can make a significant difference in how I feel. Engaging in activities like walking, swimming, or practicing yoga can help alleviate discomfort and promote flexibility.

Incorporating movement into daily routines doesn't have to be complicated or time-consuming. Small changes can lead to remarkable progress. Simple actions, like taking the stairs instead of the elevator, walking during lunch breaks, or doing light stretches while watching television, can make a big impact. One approach that has worked for me is setting specific times throughout the day to stand up and move, even if it's just for a few minutes. It's amazing how these little bursts of activity can lift my spirits and reduce tension. Finding joy in movement, no matter the form, can foster a positive mindset, creating a ripple effect that encourages even more movement. Remember, just moving your body is a victory. Every little bit counts, so take the first step and embrace the power of movement.

As you embark on this journey, it's important to listen to your body. Start slow and gradually increase the intensity of your movements as you feel comfortable. Connecting with others, whether through group classes or online communities focusing on arthritis-friendly exercises, can also provide motivation and support. Surrounding yourself with people who understand your struggles can instill a sense of camaraderie that makes movement feel less like a chore and more like an opportunity for connection and growth. Aim to make movement a regular part of your life, not just in terms of physical health but as a way to nurture your emotional well-being. Keep in mind that the key is consistency, and even the smallest step toward regular movement can lead to lasting benefits.

Gentle Exercises to Try at Home

Finding ways to stay active at home can often feel daunting, especially if you're just beginning or restarting your journey towards fitness. Gentle exercises are a great way to ease into a more active lifestyle. Consider starting with simple movements that require little to no equipment, making them easy and accessible. For instance, seated leg lifts can be done while sitting on a sturdy chair. Simply extend one leg out and hold for a few seconds before switching to the other leg. This not only strengthens your legs but also improves your mobility. Another gentle exercise is wall push-ups, where you stand a few feet from a wall and push against it. This is less intense than traditional push-ups and helps build upper body strength without straining your joints. Lastly, don't underestimate the power of stretching.

Regular stretching can improve flexibility and reduce tension, making you feel more relaxed. Try gentle neck rolls or shoulder shrugs as a way to begin incorporating movement into your daily routine without overwhelming yourself.

Promoting movement while minimizing the risk of injury or pain is crucial, especially for those who may have been inactive for a while. Listening to your body is key in this process. If you feel discomfort, it's important to adjust your movements or take a break. Start with the simplest version of each exercise and gradually increase difficulty as you become more comfortable. For instance, if leg lifts feel too challenging, try just lifting your foot a couple of inches off the ground instead. It's also beneficial to maintain good posture while exercising, as this can help prevent strain. Remember to breathe deeply and steadily; focusing on your breath can help you stay relaxed and engaged in the moment. Encouragement comes from within; remind yourself that even small steps are significant on your path to establishing a routine. Celebrate the small victories and understand that progress takes time.

Incorporating these gentle exercises into your daily life can create a positive ripple effect on your overall well-being. Try to set aside a few minutes each day for movement, even if it begins with just five minutes. A timer can help you stay committed without feeling overwhelmed. Pair your exercises with music or your favorite podcast for added motivation, making the process enjoyable. Remember, your journey towards movement doesn't need to be rigid or intense; it's about finding what feels good for you and growing from there. Keeping a journal to track your feelings and achievements during this process can also serve as a great motivator. Recognize and honor your body's capabilities and know that every effort counts towards a healthier, more active lifestyle.

Creating a Personalized Routine

Understanding your body and its unique needs is the first step towards developing a personalized exercise routine. Everyone's fitness journey is different, shaped by individual preferences, physical abilities, and goals. I remember the struggles I faced when I first started; I was unsure if I should focus on strength training or cardio, and I often felt lost among the myriad of exercise options. The real breakthrough came when I took the time to reflect on what I truly enjoyed and what my body responded to best. Sitting down and asking myself key questions was crucial. What activities did I find enjoyable? How much time could I realistically commit each week? What were my goals—weight loss, muscle gain, endurance improvement? Once I laid this foundation, it became clear how to tailor my routine.

Incorporating a variety of activities into your regimen not only keeps your workouts interesting but also helps target different muscle groups and enhances overall fitness. I found that mixing in activities such as yoga, cycling, swimming, and strength training kept me engaged. One week, I would dedicate my evenings to high-intensity interval training, and the next, I would find joy in a calming yoga session followed by a brisk walk in the park. This blend not only balanced my physical activity but allowed me to appreciate each session, rooting myself in the present moment. Experimenting with new classes or outdoor sports turned into a gateway for meeting new friends, further motivating me to remain active. Finding enjoyment in what you do is fundamental: it replaces the pressure of obligation with the pleasure of choice.

Always remember that personalizing your routine is an evolving process. It's perfectly normal to adjust as you progress or as your interests change. If you feel your motivation waning, don't hesitate to revisit those initial questions. A practical tip is to schedule a week of different activities—one day of swimming, another of hiking, perhaps a dance class or a team sport. This not only diversifies your workout but keeps your mind and body excited about what's next. Ultimately, your journey toward fitness is about discovering what works for you and embracing the path ahead with curiosity and enthusiasm.

Incorporating Stretching and Strengthening

Stretching and strengthening are more than just activities; they are essential practices for maintaining joint health. From my own experience, I have discovered that keeping my joints flexible and strong has made a significant difference in how I move each day. Stretching increases flexibility, allowing our muscles to elongate and joints to move through a greater range of motion. This increased flexibility not only aids in performance but also helps prevent injuries. On the other hand, strengthening our muscles provides the necessary support to our joints, greatly reducing stress and impact on them. It's fascinating how a regular routine of targeted stretching and strengthening can protect our bodies, making daily tasks easier and less painful.

Simple stretching techniques can easily fit into our busy lives. For instance, stretching out in the morning while still in bed can be a great way to wake up the body. Just reaching your arms overhead and extending your legs can create that pleasant feeling of stretch and release. A few minutes of neck and shoulder rolls can relieve tension that accumulates from daily activities, especially if you sit at a desk or drive a lot. During the day, try simple hamstring stretches by bending over to touch your toes or standing and lifting one leg behind you for a quadriceps stretch. These techniques take just a few moments but are extremely beneficial. Making it a habit to incorporate such stretches can prevent stiffness and maintain mobility, leading to a more vibrant and pain-free life.

Tracking Progress and Staying Motivated

Tracking progress plays a vital role in maintaining motivation and staying encouraged throughout your journey. When I first started my own path, it often felt overwhelming. However, keeping a record of my progress transformed that weight into a source of strength. Each small step, no matter how insignificant it seemed at the time, served as a reminder of how far I had come. Documenting my milestones ignited a sense of accomplishment that propelled me forward. It's important to recognize that progress isn't always linear; there will be ups and downs. But looking back at what I had achieved helped me push through the tougher days, reminding me that persistence pays off. It kept me grounded, making it easier to refocus on my goals during moments of doubt or frustration.

Using progress as a tool for setting goals and celebrating achievements can be genuinely liberating. Acknowledging the milestones along the way allowed me to set more meaningful goals. Instead of just aiming at the finish line, I started breaking my journey into smaller, actionable tasks. Each achievement, no matter how petite, became a reason to celebrate. Whether it was a personal best in a workout or simply sticking to my plan for a week, I learned to appreciate those victories. Celebrating these moments created a positive feedback loop—each celebration fueled my motivation, driving me to achieve even more. The key is to make these celebrations personal and enjoyable; they can be as simple as treating yourself to a favorite meal or sharing your achievements with a friend. By doing this, the journey transforms from a struggle into an adventure, empowering you to keep moving forward.

As you navigate your own journey, consider keeping a journal or using an app to document your progress. This practice not only helps you see how far you've come but also serves as a powerful reminder of your resiliency. Embrace the process of tracking your progress and celebrate each victory, no matter how small. With each step, remember that motivation often comes from within, ignited by the recognition of how much you can achieve. Allow your own journey to inspire you, and embrace the excitement that comes with every new goal you conquer.

Chapter 21: Stress Management

Connecting Stress and Arthritis Symptoms

Stress can feel like an unwelcome guest in our lives, especially when dealing with arthritis. The discomfort and pain already present in our joints can be exacerbated by the weight of stress. When we are stressed, our body releases hormones like cortisol, which can lead to inflammation. This inflammation is particularly troublesome for those with arthritis, as it can heighten pain and stiffness in the joints. Many of us have experienced the frustrating reality of waking up after a particularly stressful day, only to find our joints aching worse than before. It's as if stress finds a way to settle into our bodies, creating a cycle of discomfort and unease.

Understanding the connection between our mind and body is essential for managing arthritis symptoms. The mind-body connection refers to the way our mental state can influence our physical health. When we are anxious or depressed, our perception of pain can intensify, and we may become less active, which can worsen joint health. Stress often leads us to withdraw from activities we enjoy, leaving us feeling isolated and more susceptible to pain. Recognizing this connection is a powerful step. By cultivating a positive mindset and finding healthy ways to cope with stress, we can take control of our health. Techniques such as mindful breathing, meditation, or gentle physical activities, like yoga, can help soothe our minds and, in turn, alleviate some of the physical symptoms we experience.

Finding ways to reduce stress doesn't have to be a complicated endeavor. Start by incorporating small, manageable practices into your daily routine. Consider taking breaks throughout the day to stretch, breathe deeply, or simply step outside for fresh air. These moments of mindfulness can serve as an anchor, helping you navigate the tides of stress that may arise. Remember, even the smallest actions can contribute to relieving both your mind and your joints.

Mindfulness and Relaxation Techniques

Mindfulness is about being present, fully engaging with the moment and discovering peace amidst the chaos. Many of us rush through life, our minds buzzing with thoughts and worries, often missing the simple joys around us. Practicing mindfulness can significantly reduce stress and promote relaxation. When we take a moment to breathe deeply and focus on the present, we allow ourselves a break from the relentless rhythm of everyday life. This practice encourages us to acknowledge our feelings and thoughts without judgment. By fostering this kind of awareness, we can gently lessen anxiety and elevate our sense of well-being. Through mindfulness, we tune into our thoughts and emotions, realizing that they are temporary, and in doing so, we create a space for tranquility to enter our daily lives.

Incorporating mindfulness into your daily routine doesn't have to be overwhelming. Start small; perhaps as you sip your morning coffee or tea, take a moment to truly savor the taste and warmth. Notice how the cup feels in your hands and the aroma drifting upwards. Allow yourself to experience this ritual without distractions. Another easy technique is to engage in mindful breathing. Simply pause wherever you are, close your eyes if possible, and focus solely on your breath. Inhale deeply through your nose, hold for a few seconds, then exhale slowly through your mouth. This simple act, done for just a minute or two, can ground you and reduce feelings of stress. You can also practice gratitude by reflecting on three things you are thankful for each day. This not only shifts your focus from stress to appreciation but also enhances your overall mood.

Finding these little moments throughout your day to practice mindfulness can lead to significant changes over time. As you become accustomed to these techniques, you might notice improved clarity and reduced tension, which can make daily challenges feel more manageable. The key is consistency; embrace these practices without pressure. Instead of expecting immediate results, allow yourself to simply enjoy the process of being present. Over time, you may find that such mindful moments become a nourishing part of your life, leading to deeper relaxation and emotional resilience. Remember, even on the busiest days, there's always time for a brief pause to reconnect with yourself.

Creating a Peaceful Home Environment

Creating a peaceful home environment begins with the design and layout of the space. I've learned that choosing soft colors for the walls, such as light blues, greens, or warm neutrals, can significantly influence the overall mood. Natural light plays a crucial role as well; big windows that let in sunlight can lift spirits and enhance feelings of vitality. I recommend using sheer curtains to filter the light gently, creating a warm and inviting atmosphere.

Another important strategy is to declutter and organize. A cluttered space can lead to a cluttered mind, and I have often found that the act of tidying up not only clears physical space but also eases mental burdens. Reducing unnecessary items helps create breathing room, allowing you to focus on the things that truly matter. Adding personal touches, such as family photos or soothing artwork, can enhance the emotional connection to your home. Creating cozy nooks with comfortable cushions and soft throws can also provide a retreat for relaxation.

Integrating nature into your home is incredibly soothing. Incorporating indoor plants not only purifies the air but also brings a sense of tranquility. I've found that caring for plants can be a meditative practice in itself. Consider choosing low-maintenance plants like succulents or snake plants if you're unsure about your gardening skills. The gentle sound of a fountain or a bowl of smooth pebbles can also add to this calming effect. These combined elements offer not just a beautiful aesthetic but also a much-needed refuge from the chaos outside.

The environment we create at home has a profound impact on our mood and stress levels. Every color, texture, and sound contributes to how we feel in a space. Research supports the idea that certain colors can elicit psychological responses; for instance, blues and greens tend to have a calming effect, while reds and yellows can increase energy and excitement. This is something I've observed firsthand when I switched out harsh lights for softer, yellow-toned bulbs in my living area. It transformed the space into a serene retreat, helping to soothe stress after a long day.

The organization and arrangement of furniture can also affect our well-being. Open spaces that allow for smooth movement can minimize feelings of confinement and anxiety. On the other hand, a crowded space can feel overwhelming, leading to increased stress levels. I remember rearranging my living room to create a more open flow, and it made a world of difference. I began to feel lighter and more at ease within my own home.

Beyond colors and layout, the presence of noise or silence is another pivotal factor. A noisy environment can elevate stress even in the most beautifully designed space. Soundproofing can help if external noise is an issue in your area. Alternatively, consider using white noise machines or soft music to create a soothing soundscape. Even the soft rustling of leaves or distant nature sounds fosters an environment conducive to relaxation. Understanding how these elements affect our mood can empower us to create a sanctuary that cultivates peace in our lives.

To take a simple step towards creating a peaceful home, try setting aside a few minutes each day to assess how your space feels. Pay attention to what energizes you and what drains your energy. Small, intentional changes can gradually transform your environment into a calming haven.

The Role of Hobbies and Interests

Engaging in hobbies has a profound effect on our emotional and mental well-being. When I took up painting, I discovered not just a creative outlet but a sanctuary where stress melted away. With every brushstroke, worries about work deadlines and daily pressures faded into the background. Hobbies can be that special escape, allowing us to express ourselves and reconnect with our inner joy. The world can feel overwhelming at times. Finding something enjoyable, be it gardening, playing an instrument, or even woodworking, can provide a sense of accomplishment and peace that is hard to replicate elsewhere. Hobbies remind us that life is about balance and that we deserve moments of personal joy amidst our responsibilities.

Exploring interests that resonate with you can lead to unexpected sources of relaxation and fulfillment. I remember the first time I tried yoga; I was surprised by how quickly I found myself unwinding. It became a vital part of my routine, a time where I focused solely on myself and let go of the chaos around me. Whether you choose to dive deeper into a long-time passion or try something completely new, giving yourself permission to spend time on your interests can greatly enhance your overall well-being. Don't hesitate to experiment; find activities that light you up and inspire you. Finding joy doesn't require perfection; it requires the courage to try. Embrace what makes your heart smile – you'll be amazed at the difference it can make in your life.

As you explore your hobbies, remember to be kind to yourself. It's not just about the end product; it's the journey, the experience, and the joy you feel along the way. Celebrate small victories in your endeavors, whether it's finishing a painting, completing a book, or cultivating a thriving garden. Each of these moments contributes to your sense of self and helps alleviate the weariness of daily life. Prioritizing these activities can mean the difference between feeling worn out and feeling revitalized. Make it a practice to carve out time for yourself, and let your hobbies and interests lead you to a more fulfilling life. Consider dedicating just a few minutes each day to something you love – it could change everything.

Seeking Professional Help When Needed

Recognizing when to seek professional support for managing stress can often feel overwhelming, especially when faced with the challenges posed by arthritis. Stress isn't just an emotional burden; it can profoundly influence your physical health as well. When I was navigating the complexities of living with arthritis, there were moments when the frustration and fatigue seemed insurmountable. It's essential to understand that feeling this way is not a weakness but rather a signal that we might need extra help. Professional support can provide a safe space to explore these feelings, offering tools and strategies to manage not only stress but also the unique challenges that arthritis brings into our lives.

Therapeutic options can greatly complement arthritis care, helping to foster a holistic approach to well-being. Therapy isn't just about talking; it's an avenue to learn coping mechanisms that can ease the burden of daily stressors and chronic pain. Options like cognitive-behavioral therapy can help reshape negative thought patterns that worsen our perception of pain and stress. Mindfulness practices, often introduced in therapy, allow us to cultivate a sense of calm that can transform our day-to-day experiences. Whether through individual counseling or group therapy, discussing experiences with others who understand the journey can be incredibly validating. Professional help is not only a resource but a key that can unlock a healthier, more peaceful mindset.

As someone who has walked this path, I encourage you to take that first step; it's okay to ask for help. If you've been feeling overwhelmed, consider reaching out to a mental health professional or joining support groups that focus on arthritis and stress management. You deserve the support and understanding that can come from connecting with others who share your experiences. Remember, addressing emotional and mental health isn't just an option; it's an essential part of managing arthritis effectively, improving your overall quality of life.

Chapter 22: Psychological Support

The Mental Impact of Arthritis

Living with arthritis can feel like carrying a heavy burden, one that often goes unseen by the outside world. The physical pain may be apparent, but the psychological challenges are frequently overlooked. Many of us find ourselves grappling with feelings of frustration, anxiety, and even hopelessness. Each morning can bring uncertainty about how our bodies will feel, which can lead to a kind of mental fatigue that is hard to shake. It's not just the joint stiffness or swelling that affects our days, but the emotional weight that comes with adjusting to a new reality.

Isolation can become all too real, making it difficult to engage in social activities that once brought joy. Conversations may revolve around our health or we may shy away from gatherings for fear of being a burden. This can breed feelings of loneliness, as we may worry that loved ones cannot fully understand what we're experiencing. There's a sense of loss, too; the loss of spontaneity and the ability to accomplish everyday tasks without forethought or planning. Each small hurdle can compound into larger mental health issues, as we navigate our new normal.

Chronic pain can manipulate our emotions in tumultuous ways. It not only affects our physical health but seeps into our emotional landscape, leading to anxiety, depression, and mood swings. The dangerous cycle is that pain can exacerbate mental anguish, and likewise, emotional challenges can intensify physical discomfort. For some of us, moments of joy may be fleeting, overshadowed by worry about the next flare-up or the limitations imposed by our condition. It can feel like being trapped within our own bodies, a place that once felt familiar but now resembles a battleground.

Adapting to arthritis requires more than simply managing pain; it necessitates a deep dive into our own emotional health. Finding effective coping strategies can be crucial. Mindfulness, gentle exercise, or simply talking with a friend who understands can help ease the emotional burden. It's about recognizing that we are not alone in this struggle, and seeking connection can be a powerfully healing act. Cultivating patience with ourselves can be difficult, but it is essential in finding peace amidst the turbulence of chronic pain.

In times of struggle, remember to reach out for support and share your experiences. A support group or a mental health professional can provide valuable insights and guidance. Each day may bring new challenges, but it's vital to acknowledge the small victories along the way. Practicing gratitude for the good moments, no matter how brief, can make the journey more bearable and help spark motivation for the days ahead.

Coping Strategies for Emotional Well-Being

Coping strategies play a vital role in building emotional resilience. When faced with life's inevitable challenges, it becomes essential to cultivate a toolkit of strategies that can help navigate through difficult times. Consider engaging in physical activities such as walking, running, or even dancing. These activities not only boost your mood through the release of endorphins but also provide a sense of accomplishment and purpose. Finding a creative outlet can also be incredibly healing. Whether it's painting, writing, or playing an instrument, expressing your thoughts and feelings through art can help alleviate stress and promote emotional clarity. Connecting with others is another powerful coping strategy. Surrounding yourself with supportive friends or family members can create a buffer against tough times, offering not just emotional support but also different perspectives on issues. Engaging in community service or volunteering can also foster a deeper sense of connection and fulfillment, helping shift focus away from personal struggles to the needs of others. Remember, there is no one-size-fits-all approach to coping; exploring different strategies will help you discover what resonates best with you.

As we navigate challenges, self-compassion and mindfulness become two vital ingredients in promoting emotional well-being. Embracing self-compassion means treating ourselves with kindness when we encounter setbacks instead of being our own harshest critics. It allows us to acknowledge our struggles without judgment, creating space for healing and positive change. When we practice self-compassion, we learn to understand that everyone faces difficulties and that it's okay to not be okay sometimes. Mindfulness practices, such as meditation and grounding exercises, can help anchor us in the present. These techniques encourage us to observe our thoughts and feelings without getting overwhelmed by them. When we are mindful, we can better respond to stressors rather than react impulsively. This blend of self-compassion and mindfulness not only helps us create a nurturing inner dialogue but also equips us to handle challenges with greater ease. Starting small, like taking a few moments each day to breathe deeply or jot down what we are grateful for, can pave the way for significant changes in our emotional landscape.

Building emotional resilience is a journey that requires patience and practice. One useful tip is to make a commitment to check in with yourself regularly. Set aside a moment each day, perhaps in the morning or just before bed, to reflect on your feelings and thoughts without judgment. This practice not only helps foster self-awareness, but it also enables you to identify potential stressors before they escalate. As you begin to recognize your emotional patterns, you can tailor your coping strategies more effectively. It's about understanding that emotional well-being is like a muscle—the more you care for it, the stronger it becomes. Embrace the process, and remember that every step you take toward enhancing your emotional resilience is a step worth celebrating.

Importance of Therapy and Counseling

Living with arthritis can often feel like an uphill battle, with its relentless physical symptoms often accompanied by an emotional toll that is hard to articulate. Beyond the discomfort of swollen joints and fatigue, there can be an undercurrent of sadness, frustration, and isolation. Therapy provides a space to explore these feelings in a supportive environment, helping individuals process their experiences and find ways to cope with the challenges arthritis presents. It is not uncommon to face moments of deep emotional pain, and sharing these moments with a trained professional can bring clarity and comfort. Through talk therapy, many learn valuable coping strategies that not only make managing pain more bearable but also enhance their overall quality of life. The compassionate guidance offered by therapists can help individuals navigate the complex emotions tied to their condition, cultivating resilience and hope.

Integrating professional support into your care plan is not just an option; it can be a crucial step toward emotional well-being. A therapist can serve as a partner in your journey, providing a fresh perspective and sustainable coping mechanisms. Whether it's through cognitive-behavioral therapy that challenges negative thought patterns or mindfulness techniques that promote relaxation and acceptance, professional help can be invaluable. Many individuals might feel uncertain about reaching out for help, but acknowledging the need for support is a courageous step. Just as your physical health requires medical attention, so too does your emotional health. Finding the right therapist who understands arthritis can make a significant difference, empowering you to reclaim your life and face each day with renewed strength.

Incorporating therapy into your routine can be as essential as any medication in your treatment plan. Consider starting with just one session to see how it feels. It's about finding a safe space to express yourself and process your journey, and you don't have to do it alone. Establishing a connection with a therapist can offer insights that lead to a more comprehensive understanding of your experiences. Ultimately, prioritizing your mental health alongside your physical health creates a more holistic approach to living with arthritis. Take that first step, and commit to nurturing both your body and your mind.

Building a Support Network

Having a supportive network of friends, family, and peers can make a world of difference in our lives. It's in the small moments when we feel overwhelmed or uncertain that we really see the true value of these connections. The warmth of a friend's reassuring words, the comfort of a family member's embrace, or the encouraging nod of a peer who understands our journey can propel us to face challenges with renewed strength. I remember a time in my life when I felt utterly alone, grappling with self-doubt and fear. It was only when I opened up to a few close friends that I realized I wasn't alone in my struggles. They shared their own experiences, which made me feel validated and less isolated. Building and nurturing these relationships is not just beneficial; it's essential for our emotional and mental well-being. These bonds remind us that we belong, that we are valued, and that our feelings matter. They provide a safety net, allowing us to take risks and pursue our goals with the knowledge that we have a cheering squad behind us.

To enhance connection and communication with our loved ones, we can adopt a few intentional strategies. First and foremost, being present when with others is crucial. This means putting down our phones and genuinely engaging in conversations, listening actively, and responding from the heart. I've found that when I make an effort to really listen, my relationships deepen in ways I never expected. Asking open-ended questions can also encourage deeper dialogues and shared reflections. It's these conversations that often lead to mutual support and understanding. Creating regular touchpoints with friends and family—be it through texts, phone calls, or scheduled meet-ups—can significantly bolster these relationships. When we make the effort to check in, we not only strengthen our connections but also show that we care. Lastly, sharing experiences, whether it's through joint hobbies, attending workshops, or simply exploring new places together, strengthens the ties that bind us. These shared memories and adventures become the threads that weave our lives together more closely.

Self-Care Practices for Mental Health

Incorporating self-care routines that nourish mental and emotional health is essential for everyone seeking balance and well-being. Think about those moments when you feel overwhelmed; it's all too easy to forget about yourself amidst responsibilities and stressors. One practical step I've found helpful is establishing a morning routine that includes mindfulness or meditation. Setting aside just ten minutes to focus on your breath and be present can create a calm foundation for the day. You can also think about journaling your thoughts or feelings as a way to process emotions and thoughts. Pouring your heart out onto paper can be incredibly relieving, helping you to make sense of what you're feeling and why. Creative activities, like drawing, painting, or even gardening, can serve as wonderful outlets for expressing yourself and nurturing your soul. This gives you space to explore your emotions without judgment, allowing you to reconnect with what truly matters to you.

On the journey to resilience, practical self-care techniques can make all the difference. Engaging in physical activity is a powerful way to boost your mood and energy levels. It doesn't have to be an intense workout; leisurely walks in nature can provide the fresh air and change of scenery you need to clear your mind. It's fascinating how simply moving your body can release endorphins, which are natural mood lifters. Building connections with others is equally vital. Sharing experiences with friends or family can create a support network that fosters resilience. Even a phone call or text message can remind you that you're not alone in your struggles. Additionally, practicing gratitude can shift your perspective tremendously. Taking a moment each day to reflect on things you're thankful for can cultivate a more positive mindset, enhancing your ability to face challenges with grace.

It's important to remember that self-care isn't selfish; it's crucial for maintaining your overall health. Making time for yourself might feel indulgent, but it's an investment in your well-being. Try setting boundaries with work or other responsibilities to carve out moments dedicated to self-care, even if it's just a few minutes here and there. Think of it as filling your cup so that you can show up fully for others in your life. Experiment with different self-care strategies until you find what resonates with you. Most importantly, give yourself permission to prioritize your mental health without guilt. Developing these supportive habits can pave the way for a healthier mindset and a more fulfilled life. Embrace the journey of self-care; it's one of the most important gifts you can give yourself.

Chapter 23: Long-term Home Planning

Future-proofing Your Home

Making long-term adjustments to your home is a proactive way to ensure not only safety but also comfort as you navigate through various life stages. Small changes can lead to significant improvements in how you experience your living space. Start by evaluating areas that could pose a risk or discomfort. For instance, lighting is often overlooked, but brighter, well-placed lights can make a world of difference in reducing hazards, especially in hallways and staircases. Consider installing motion sensor lights to enhance convenience and eliminate the need to fumble in the dark. Additionally, if you have stairs, think about investing in sturdy handrails or even a stairlift if needed. Remember, it's not just about aesthetics; it's about creating an environment where you can feel secure and at ease. Making your home a safe haven should be a priority.

As we think about the future, it's essential to anticipate our needs, especially as we age. Maintaining independence is not just about mobility; it's about creating a space that supports your lifestyle choices. Start imagining how your daily routines might change in the years to come. Will you need grab bars in the bathroom? Perhaps a shower that doesn't require stepping over a high ledge? Planning these changes now can save both time and stress later on. Consider using smart home technology, like voice-activated assistants, which can help control lights, thermostats, and even security systems. This way, you maintain the control and independence you desire without compromising safety. Tailoring your home to your evolving needs is an empowering step towards ensuring you can continue to thrive in your space.

Being proactive about future-proofing your home is not just about preserving physical spaces but nurturing your emotional well-being. When your environment feels naturally supportive of your journey, it fosters a sense of freedom and confidence in everyday activities. One practical tip to get started is to compile a list of changes that would enhance your daily life. This could include everything from the type of furniture you have to the accessibility of your kitchen. By framing your home as an ongoing project that evolves with you, you affirm the importance of your needs and aspirations. Your home can and should be a reflection of your life, ensuring that as the years go by, you continue to feel comfortable, safe, and inspired within its walls.

Renovations for Aging in Place

Creating a home that embraces aging in place means designing a space that promotes comfort, safety, and accessibility. It starts with understanding and anticipating the various challenges that can come with getting older. Simple renovations can make a profound difference. Consider widening doorways and hallways to accommodate mobility aids, eliminating barriers like steps, and choosing non-slip flooring to reduce the risk of falls. Installing grab bars in showers and beside the toilet can offer reassurance as well. Additionally, adding a walk-in shower rather than a traditional bath can transform a potentially hazardous environment into a haven of ease. Think about adjusting the height of light switches and outlets for greater accessibility, and make sure to have plenty of bright, even lighting throughout your home. These small upgrades can create a supportive environment that fosters independence and safety.

Planning for features that enhance ease and reduce risks requires a proactive approach. Installing night lights can illuminate paths during the dark hours, preventing accidents in the middle of the night. Lever-style faucets are easier to operate than knobs, and thermostatic shower valves can help avoid scalding. You might want to consider smart technology, such as voice-activated assistants or automatic lighting systems, which can simplify daily routines. When thinking about the kitchen, lower countertops can make cooking and food preparation more accessible, along with easy-to-reach cabinets. It's also beneficial to create spaces that encourage movement without falls—like providing ample room around furniture, removing clutter, and ensuring everyone can easily get to essential areas in their home. Making these thoughtful changes not only contributes to a safer living environment but also nurtures a sense of dignity and empowerment.

As you embark on these renovations, involve family members or trusted friends who understand your needs and can provide valuable insights. Their support can ensure the renovations are not just functional but also reflective of your personal style and preferences. Every change you make is a step toward preserving your lifestyle and enhancing your quality of life. Always remember: it's not just about the physical changes but also about fostering an emotional connection to your home. A welcoming, safe, and accessible space can significantly enrich your overall well-being as you navigate the journey of aging in place.

Budgeting for Home Modifications

Creating a budget for necessary home modifications can be a daunting task, especially when navigating the emotional aspects of adapting your living environment. It requires a thoughtful approach and strategies that not only prioritize your financial health but also address your unique needs. Start by assessing your overall financial situation, including income, savings, and any potential funding sources such as grants or government programs specifically designed for home accessibility. Consider setting realistic spending limits and identifying areas where you can cut costs or save money that can be directed towards modifications. Flexible options like creating a phased plan for your renovations can also be beneficial. This allows you to make essential changes now and spread the cost over time, giving you the freedom to adapt without overwhelming financial pressure.

When it comes to prioritizing modifications, it's essential to identify which changes can bring the most significant benefits to your daily life. Think about modifications that enhance your safety, mobility, or independence. For example, adding grab bars in the bathroom or widening doorways may seem small, but they can drastically improve accessibility and comfort. Engage with professionals who specialize in home modifications to understand which changes can have the most impact and how to execute them efficiently. It's not just about the modifications themselves but the overall quality of life they bring. Consider your personal routines and activities; if cooking is a cherished interest, investing in a kitchen remodel that accommodates your needs could be a priority. By focusing on the modifications that resonate most with you and your lifestyle, you create a home that not only feels safe but also supports your passions and interests.

Budgeting and home modifications don't have to be a stressful experience. Keeping track of your expenses in a simple spreadsheet can help you visualize your spending and plan ahead. Finding community resources or online forums where others share their experiences can also provide crucial support and insight. Remember, every small change adds up, and finding joy in the process of adapting your home can empower you to create the living space you've always wanted. You've got this, one step at a time.

Consulting Professionals for Advice

Seeking advice from experts on effective home modifications can feel daunting, especially when you're navigating the complexities of making your living space work better for you. Whether you're dealing with accessibility issues, aesthetic changes, or simply searching for improved functionality, I encourage you to reach out to professionals who specialize in these areas. Consultants, architects, interior designers, and occupational therapists are armed with knowledge and experience that can transform your home into a place that not only meets your needs but inspires you to thrive. Imagine walking into a room that is tailored just for you, crafted with intention to bring out the best in your daily life. This transformation begins with asking the right questions and seeking out those who can guide you through the process.

There is a wealth of resources available for professional assistance that can open doors to new ideas and possibilities. Online platforms and community groups offer a robust network where individuals share experiences and recommendations. Local workshops and seminars can also be great places to connect with industry professionals who are eager to share their insights. Additionally, utilizing professional directories or freelance platforms allows you to find consultants who match your specific needs, whether it's a simple design overhaul or a significant structural change. Don't underestimate the power of social media and forums—these can be valuable places for gathering knowledge and inspiration. Every small step in seeking expert advice takes you closer to a space where you can feel more comfortable and empowered.

As you embark on this journey, remember that asking for help is a sign of strength, not weakness. It can be the key to unlocking a home environment that truly supports your aspirations. Embrace the knowledge of those who have walked this path before you, and don't hesitate to reach out for guidance. Connecting with the right professionals can open up new avenues of creativity and practicality that you might not have considered. Take the first step today by jotting down the specific changes you envision—this will help you articulate your needs clearly when consulting with experts. Your dream home is within reach, and the professionals you consult can help guide you on that journey.

Evaluating Your Progress Over Time

As you start to adapt your home to better suit your needs, it's essential to have a clear strategy for monitoring the effectiveness of those changes over time. Begin by keeping a journal or a digital log where you can note your experiences with each adaptation. Write down what works well and what feels comfortable, as well as any challenges you encounter. Engaging regularly in this reflection allows you to track patterns and identify areas needing improvement. Consider setting aside time weekly or monthly to review these notes. Be honest with yourself; this is your journey, and it's important to recognize both successes and setbacks. Observing how adaptations influence your daily life can also serve as a powerful motivator, reminding you of how far you've come.

Regularly evaluate physical elements in your environment, such as the ease of getting in and out of your home, the accessibility of your kitchen, or the comfort of your bathroom setup. Invite trusted friends or family members for an outside perspective; they might notice things you overlook. Conducting this assessment in a compassionate way can be freeing, as it helps you embrace the changes rather than feel trapped by them. Taking a few moments each day to reflect on how safe and comfortable you feel in your own space is crucial. Use this self-awareness to discover what might need to be adjusted. When adaptations feel daunting or inconvenient, it's okay to ask for help – whether from a professional or someone close to you who can offer support.

Once you've gathered insights about your home adaptations and how they serve you, the next step is to be willing to adjust your plans as necessary. Flexibility is a key element in creating a living space that truly supports your needs. For instance, if you've added grab bars but find they don't provide enough support or are located awkwardly, don't hesitate to reposition them or consult with an expert about different options. Trial and error is part of this process, and every adjustment you make is a step toward greater safety and comfort.

It's also helpful to stay informed about new technologies or products designed for accessibility. There may be innovations you hadn't considered that could significantly improve your daily experiences. Reach out to community resources or forums where you can exchange ideas with others navigating similar challenges. This communal sharing fosters an environment of support and encouragement, reminding you that you're not alone. Rather than feeling overwhelmed by potential changes, view each adjustment as an opportunity to optimize your living space, making it more enjoyable and suited to your life.

Lastly, prioritize self-compassion throughout this journey. Recognizing that adapting your home is a continual process will help to ease any pressure you may place on yourself. Celebrate the small victories, and remind yourself that every proactive step you take contributes to your overall quality of life. If you're feeling uncertain about a particular change, take the time to discuss it with someone you trust to gain a fresh perspective. Embrace the process of evolving and adjusting, knowing it leads you closer to the safety and comfort you deserve.

Chapter 24: Collaborating with Professionals

When to Seek Professional Help

Recognizing the right moment to enlist professional help can often feel overwhelming, especially when managing arthritis. There are signs that can guide your decision. If you notice that your pain is becoming more persistent or severe, or if routine tasks are increasingly challenging, it may be a signal that you need additional support. Understand that you don't have to face this alone. Many individuals often push through discomfort, thinking they can manage on their own or that their situation might improve with time. However, early intervention can be crucial in preventing further complications and improving your quality of life. Don't hesitate to seek assistance when the pain begins to interfere with daily activities or impacts your emotional well-being. Listening to your body and recognizing when a comforting voice or expert guidance is needed can be the first step towards regaining control.

Understanding the benefits of professional support in managing arthritis is key to your journey. Professionals like rheumatologists, physical therapists, and occupational therapists have specialized knowledge that can make a significant difference in your treatment plan. They can offer tailored strategies and interventions that not only help alleviate pain but also improve mobility and enhance everyday function. For instance, a physical therapist can guide you through exercises that strengthen your joints, while a rheumatologist can provide medication options that alleviate inflammation. Moreover, seeking help is not just about physical treatment; it also includes emotional support. Professional counselors or support groups can provide safe spaces to share your feelings and experiences, helping you cope with the emotional toll arthritis can sometimes take. This multifaceted approach can foster a sense of optimism, helping you create a balanced life despite the challenges of arthritis.

Pay attention to the signs your body gives you, and remember that reaching out for professional help is a sign of strength, not weakness. Whether it's scheduling that long-postponed appointment or simply discussing your symptoms with someone who understands, taking action can lead to relief and empowerment. With the right support, not only can you navigate the complexities of arthritis, but you can also reclaim joy in your everyday life.

Types of Professionals to Consult

When navigating the challenges of arthritis, understanding the types of professionals available for support can significantly enhance your journey towards managing pain and improving your quality of life. Various specialists can play vital roles in your care, ensuring you receive a holistic approach that addresses both physical and emotional needs. From rheumatologists who specialize in diagnosing and treating arthritis to physical therapists who can tailor exercise regimens to your specific limitations, consulting with the right professionals can make a world of difference. Occupational therapists can help you adapt your daily living activities to minimize strain while dietitians can offer insights on nutrition that may help manage inflammation. Each of these professionals brings unique skills to the table, and it's essential to see them not just as practitioners but as partners who can empower you in your journey.

Identifying the right experts to support you involves understanding your personal needs and recognizing when to seek help. Consider reaching out to a rheumatologist if you're experiencing joint pain, swelling, or fatigue, as they can provide a comprehensive assessment and develop an effective treatment plan. Physical therapists can also be invaluable allies, guiding you through exercises designed to strengthen your muscles while protecting your joints. Meanwhile, don't overlook the benefits of working with a mental health professional, especially when dealing with the emotional toll arthritis can take. An empathetic therapist can help you cope with feelings of frustration or sadness, offering coping strategies that resonate with your personal experience. By forming a support network of qualified professionals, you can better navigate the ups and downs of arthritis.

As you consider who to consult, remember that these professionals are here to help you regain control over your life. They understand the complexities of living with arthritis and can provide individualized care that addresses your unique situation. Don't hesitate to communicate your concerns or ask questions; a good professional will appreciate your input and work with you to find the best solutions. Keep in mind that the journey may not always be easy, but by surrounding yourself with the right support team, you can cultivate resilience. A practical tip is to maintain a journal of your symptoms, questions, and any progress you notice. This not only helps you articulate your experience during appointments but also empowers you to actively participate in your treatment plan.

Creating a Plan with Healthcare Providers

Creating a care plan with your healthcare providers is vital for achieving your health goals. When we take the time to communicate openly about our concerns and aspirations, we are building a partnership that can greatly enhance our well-being. It's not just about visiting the doctor and receiving a prescription; it's about having a thorough understanding of our health status, what we want to achieve, and the best ways to get there. Imagine sitting down with your doctor, discussing your everyday challenges, and together developing a strategy that respects your lifestyle and meets your needs. This collaborative approach not only fosters trust but also empowers you to take charge of your health.

As we engage in this process, we can identify specific health goals, whether it's managing a chronic condition, improving fitness, or achieving mental clarity. These personalized goals are essential, as they give us something tangible to work towards, making the journey feel real and achievable. A care plan is more than just a document; it's a roadmap that outlines the steps you need to take, the resources available to you, and the milestones that indicate progress. It provides clarity and direction, reducing feelings of overwhelm that often accompany health challenges.

Your role in this process is crucial. Actively participating in your health management can be the difference between feeling helpless and feeling empowered. Embrace the opportunity to ask questions, voice your concerns, and share personal experiences. Doing so not only informs your healthcare provider about what matters most to you but also strengthens your own understanding of your health journey. Take the initiative to research your health condition, explore treatment options, and understand the rationale behind each recommendation. The more informed you are, the more confident you will feel in making decisions about your health.

One practical tip is to maintain a health journal. Documenting your symptoms, moods, and lifestyle changes can provide valuable insights during your healthcare visits. This simple tool can help guide discussions with your healthcare providers, ensuring that your concerns are addressed and your journey remains focused.

Engagement with Occupational Therapists

Understanding the role of occupational therapists in increasing independence is vital for individuals facing challenges in their everyday lives. Occupational therapists work closely with clients to assess their unique needs and establish personalized plans that target specific goals. These professionals are not just experts in health; they often have a deep understanding of the practical challenges that come with various physical or mental health concerns. They help you discover new strategies to tackle the activities you used to do effortlessly. Their empathetic approach makes it easier to talk about your struggles, creating a supportive environment where you can openly express your needs and aspirations. Through their guidance, you can find pathways that lead to greater independence, reclaiming aspects of your life that may have felt lost for some time.

Therapy can significantly assist with daily tasks and activities, reshaping how you interact with your environment. Whether it's learning adaptive techniques to complete household chores or finding new ways to engage in hobbies and social activities, occupational therapists equip you with essential skills. They encourage the use of assistive devices, which can make a world of difference in your daily routine. For example, simple modifications in your home or routines can transform daunting tasks into manageable ones. When faced with the challenge of cooking, for instance, an occupational therapist may help you break down the process into smaller, achievable steps, or suggest adaptive utensils that ease your experience in the kitchen. This kind of personalized assistance fosters a sense of accomplishment, helping you to build confidence and autonomy.

Engaging with an occupational therapist is more than just therapy; it's a partnership centered around your journey to independence. As you work together, you'll likely find that the goals you set are not just about what you can do but also about who you want to be. The process can be emotional, but the support you receive makes the journey easier. Remember, it's okay to ask for help, and taking the step to engage with an occupational therapist may be one of the best choices you make. Finding joy in small successes can be incredibly motivating, and they often suggest keeping a journal to celebrate those victories. Documenting your progress serves as a reminder of your resilience and can provide encouragement on tougher days.

Home Consultants for Upgrades and Design

Finding comfort and ease in our homes becomes increasingly important when living with arthritis. Home consultants who specialize in arthritis-friendly design focus on creating spaces that cater to our unique needs. These professionals understand the challenges we face daily, from managing pain to dealing with stiffness. They look at every angle, offering practical solutions like zero-threshold shower entries, wider doorways to accommodate mobility aids, and ergonomic furniture that minimizes strain. The options are broad, and consultants can guide us toward the right features that make home life not just bearable, but truly enjoyable.

The main advantage of seeking professional input is that these consultants bring a wealth of knowledge tailored to creating accessible spaces. They can turn our personal preferences into tangible designs, ensuring that our homes reflect who we are while being functional and accommodating. Professional consultants don't just modify rooms; they rethink layouts and utilize materials that enhance comfort. For instance, they might suggest softer flooring to reduce stress on joints or innovative storage solutions to minimize bending and reaching. These enhancements empower us to navigate our spaces independently and safely, reducing the risk of falls or injury. Working with professionals often leads to solutions we might overlook, ensuring our homes are true havens of comfort and accessibility.

Investing time with a home consultant can seem daunting at first, but engaging in this process can yield incredible benefits. Look for individuals or firms that showcase their experience with arthritis-friendly designs. These specialists will help translate your needs into a cohesive plan that transforms your space into an accommodating environment. Remember, the goal is to create a living area where moving about feels effortless. It's not just about making adjustments; it's about reclaiming the joy of being home. Don't hesitate to explore every possibility, as each thoughtful decision adds up to a far more comfortable and enriching life. Seek out advice, stay informed, and never underestimate the difference a well-designed home can make.

Chapter 25: Conclusion and Next Steps

Recap of Key Changes

This book has journeyed through crucial transformations that many of us might experience in our lives. We talked about embracing vulnerability, shifting mindsets, and cultivating resilience. Each chapter unfolded a tapestry of insights designed to empower you. The importance of reconnecting with your inner strength surfaced repeatedly, showing how vital it is to truly understand and accept ourselves. We explored the means to foster healthier relationships, both with ourselves and those around us, and shared stories of growth and self-discovery that underscore these changes. Life isn't static; each new perspective or practice we adopt creates ripples across our reality, altering our everyday experiences and forging paths we once thought unreachable.

As you reflect on these modifications, consider how they might reshape various aspects of your life. What does embracing vulnerability mean for you personally? Imagine stepping into your authenticity, shedding the mask imposed by society. Feel the transformative power of this shift and envision how it can enhance your interactions and self-perception. Think about the potential for deeper connections with family, friends, and with your own aspirations. Each small change can generate significant outcomes— notice how gratitude can brighten your outlook or how a simple adjustment in mindset can help you tackle life's challenges. Your journey, shaped by the insights gleaned from this book, is not just about personal growth but about thriving in all areas of life.

As you move forward, remember that reflection is just the beginning. Take a moment each day to integrate these lessons into your life. Whether it's through journaling your thoughts, setting new intentions, or simply checking in with yourself, these practices can bolster your commitment to change. Tiny steps taken consistently lead to profound transformations—never underestimate the power of small actions over time. Embrace this ongoing process with an open heart and a curious mind, and observe how it brings not just changes but enriches your journey.

Setting Goals for Improvement

Establishing realistic goals for your health and home environment is not just a task; it's an essential journey that requires mindfulness and compassion towards yourself. It's vital to take a step back and assess where you currently stand, both physically and in your living space. Start by identifying specific areas that feel overwhelming or in need of improvement. Maybe your diet has become routine, or your living room feels cluttered. By breaking down these larger concerns into smaller, manageable goals, you create a roadmap for yourself. Instead of telling yourself to eat healthier overall, consider starting with one meatless meal each week. If your living space feels chaotic, you might choose to declutter one corner of your home each week. Each of these smaller goals becomes a stepping stone, making the process feel less daunting and more achievable.

Celebrating small achievements along this journey is crucial. Every time you accomplish a goal, no matter how minor it may seem, give yourself permission to feel proud. These moments of recognition can work wonders for your motivation. When I decided to take a weekly walk instead of watching TV, I felt a surge of accomplishment each time I returned home, breathless and exhilarated by my small victory. It's important to acknowledge these milestones—whether it's treating yourself to your favorite healthy snack after a week of good eating or simply taking a moment to feel grateful for a clean space. This practice not only boosts your confidence but also reinforces a positive mindset. Remember, progress is not merely about the end results but about the journey and the small victories along the way. Every step forward is a reason to celebrate.

As you embark on this path of improvement, take a moment to reflect on what you truly value. Setting goals aligned with your passions and interest not only brings clarity but ensures your commitment to see them through. This alignment makes all the difference when faced with temptation or obstacles. Keep a journal to document your aspirations and achievements. This will not only serve as a reference for progress but also as motivation when the going gets tough. Always remind yourself that improvement is a personal journey; it's okay to progress at your own pace. Each small step contributes to a larger, more fulfilling lifestyle.

Maintaining a Positive Outlook

Maintaining a positive mindset is essential, especially when life throws challenges our way. I've experienced moments where everything seemed to fall apart, and it was tempting to succumb to despair. In those tough times, I learned that a positive outlook is not about ignoring difficulties but about choosing to confront them with hope. This shift in perspective allowed me to navigate obstacles rather than be crushed by them. Acknowledging the challenges is the first step; embracing a belief that something better lies ahead keeps us moving forward. Research shows that a positive mindset can improve our overall health, increase our resilience, and lead to a more fulfilling life. Every time we choose hope over despair, we not only uplift ourselves but also inspire those around us to do the same.

Fostering hope and resilience takes practice and intention. One effective strategy is to cultivate gratitude. Each day, I try to reflect on three things I'm thankful for, no matter how small they may seem. This simple act shifts my focus from what I lack to what I have, bringing clarity and perspective. Another powerful tool is surrounding ourselves with positive influences. I noticed that spending time with encouraging friends and family fuels my own sense of hope. Engaging in activities that bring joy or passion, whether it's a hobby or physical exercise, also plays a crucial role in building resilience. Finally, it's important to set small, achievable goals. When I accomplish these mini-milestones, I feel a sense of progress that encourages me to tackle larger challenges. By combining these practices, we can effectively nurture a mindset that thrives even in tough times.

Remember, hope is not a passive state; it's something we can actively cultivate, and each step, no matter how small, brings us closer to a brighter future.

Write down a few things that inspire hope for you and share them with someone close to you. This small act of connection can create a ripple effect, fostering a supportive environment where positivity thrives.

Resources for Ongoing Support

Finding the right resources and support can make a significant difference in your journey with arthritis. There are numerous organizations dedicated to helping those who battle this condition, offering everything from educational materials to practical advice. The Arthritis Foundation is a cornerstone resource; they provide valuable information, support groups, and even fitness programs designed specifically for people with arthritis. Their website is a treasure trove of resources to help sufferers better understand their condition and connect with others facing similar challenges.

Another valuable organization is the National Rheumatoid Arthritis Society, which focuses on advancing treatment options while also providing a strong support network for patients and their families. Connecting with organizations like these can empower you to take charge of your health, providing you with tools and strategies to improve your quality of life. Many local communities also have support groups, which can be helpful as they create a space to share personal experiences, discuss coping strategies, and find that you are not alone in this journey.

Engaging with your community is not just about finding support; it's about giving support as well. Sharing your experiences, whether through formal support groups or informal gatherings, creates bonds that can uplift and inspire others who may be struggling. When you reach out, it can open doors to friendships and social connections that enrich your life and alleviate some of the isolation that often comes with chronic illness. Local events, workshops, or even online forums can be great places to connect with others who understand what you're going through and can offer empathy and encouragement. By becoming part of a community, you can foster a sense of belonging that brings hope and motivation into your day-to-day life.

Consider making a habit of seeking out at least one resource or community engagement opportunity each week. It could be as simple as attending a local event or reaching out to someone for a chat. Taking small steps can lead to greater mental and emotional support and can help you navigate your journey with arthritis more smoothly.

Encouragement to Take Action

It's time to take charge of your life and implement the changes that resonate deep within you. You might have felt a stirring in your heart while reading this book, a call from your innermost self urging you to pursue the life you've always dreamed of. Every great transformation begins with a single step. The insights and tools you have learned are waiting for you to put them into practice. Change can often be daunting, but it's essential to remember that it is also a magnificent opportunity for growth. Imagine waking up each day with purpose, feeling energized by the possibilities that lie ahead. Now is the moment to translate your aspirations into actions. By committing to change, you are choosing to believe in yourself and the power you hold to shape your destiny.

As you stand on the precipice of this journey, take a moment to visualize the positive transformation awaiting you. You have the potential for growth, healing, and renewal—in every aspect of your life. Each decision you make, no matter how small, acts as a building block toward your dreams. Trust that you have the strength to rise above challenges and the resilience to keep moving forward, even when the path becomes unclear. Goals can be achieved. Relationships can flourish. Your inner peace can become a reality. Picture yourself in a future where you have embraced the changes you dared to make; it is within your reach. Every effort you invest in this process will yield substantial rewards, propelling you toward fulfillment and joy.

To kickstart this transformative journey, take a moment each day to reflect on one action you can take that aligns with your new intentions. Whether it's journaling your thoughts, exercising, or reaching out to a supportive friend, these small steps can create a ripple effect of positive change. Consistency is key, and each time you prioritize these actions, you reinforce your commitment to growth. Start visualizing the person you wish to become, and trust that you are capable of making that vision a reality.

Thank You for Your Purchase

Congratulation on completing

Adapting Your Home: Simple Changes to Reduce

Arthritis Risk

Please look out for our other eBooks on

Self-care coming soon!

LA Smith

Made in United States
Troutdale, OR
07/12/2025

32867955R00116